LIVE FULLY, LOVE FREELY
WITH MENTAL ILLNESS

60-DAY DEVOTIONAL

Jared Cash

Live Fully, Love Freely with Mental Illness: 60-Day Devotional

Copyright © 2021 by Jared Cash

Library of Congress Cataloging-in-Publication Data

Cash, Jared, 1992 –

Live Fully, Love Freely with Mental Illness: 60-Day Devotional

p. cm.

ISBN: 978-0-578-91139-7 (ebook)

ISBN: 978-0-578-91138-0 (Soft cover)

1. Devotional calendars. 2. Devotional literature, English.

Printed in the United States of America

DEDICATION

For Jessica, Juliette, and Adeline.

Jessica, you have been in the trenches with me during the highest of highs and the lowest of lows. You push me daily to be the man that God created me to be. You help me see the beauty in life. You truly are my better half.

Juliette and Adeline, you provide more joy in my life than you will ever know. I am incredibly proud to be your dad. I pray you always pursue Jesus passionately.

I love you three with all of my heart.

ACKNOWLEDGEMENTS

To my mom and dad, you have been there since the beginning of my journey with mental illness and were two of my biggest supporters in writing this book. Thank you for never giving up on me. You are the best parents I could ever ask for and two of my best friends.

Jordan and Corrie, your constant support and encouragement has helped me more than you will ever know. I am extremely blessed to have you two in my corner cheering me on. I'm thankful for my little man, Elliott, too.

Matt, K-Mo, K-Mac, Josh, and Nolan, you have been the five most solid friendships these past years as I navigated through life and mental illness. Your continued encouragement kept me going on the days I needed it the most.

John and Stephen, you both helped me see Jesus in the middle of my brokenness. You were there for me in my most confusing season and for that I am forever grateful. Thank you for allowing God to pour out of you into my life.

Kay and Dr. Earp, you both helped me understand more about mental illness and provided numerous tools to help me manage it. I would not be in the place I am now without you.

Pastor David, Billy, Steve, and Mike, my transition into a time of healing would not have been possible without you four men. You listened, cared, and supported me in every way possible. Thank you for loving my family and I so well.

Contents

Acknowledgements vii

Introduction 1

Day 1: One is the Loneliest Number 3

Day 2: Barely Reaching for Coffee 5

Day 3: Where is the Love? 7

Day 4: It's Okay to Not Be Okay 9

Day 5: Let Go of Embarrassment 11

Day 6: Counting Sheep 13

Day 7: Start the Day Right 17

Day 8: Benefits of Exercise 19

Day 9: Brain Fuel 21

Day 10: The Pace of Life 23

Day 11: The Greatest Decision 25

Day 12: Burdens of the Day 27

Day 13: Chains 29

Day 14: Where Can I Turn? 31

Day 15: Your Soul Needs Worship 33

Day 16: Hope for the Hopeless 35

Day 17: When Anxiety Attacks 37

Day 18: Be Still and Allow God to be God 39

Day 19: Choosing Love 41

Day 20: I Need Answers 43

Day 21: East to West 45

Day 22: Bottle of Tears 47

Day 23: Victory in the Midst of Pain 49

Day 24: View of God 51

Day 25: God's Love Note 53

Day 26: Shine a Light 55
Day 27: Hide and Seek 57
Day 28: Hearing the Whisper 59
Day 29: A Healthy, Happy You 63
Day 30: What's Fear Got to Do with It? 65
Day 31: Wrong Questions, Wrong Answers? 69
Day 32: Thankfulness 71
Day 33: Don't Stay in Isolation 73
Day 34: Snowflakes and Fingerprints 77
Day 35: Communication, Communication, Communication . 79
Day 36: Sunrise to Sunset 81
Day 37: A Time of Healing 83
Day 38: I Know I Need to Say No 85
Day 39: Joy, Joy, Joy 87
Day 40: Taking Refuge 89
Day 41: Peace of God 91
Day 42: I Worry That I Worry Too Much 93
Day 43: Is Pain a Waste? 95
Day 44: Created for the Valley 97
Day 45: Usefulness Through Brokenness 99
Day 46: The Sun Still Shines 101
Day 47: Fight or Flight 103
Day 48: Never-Ending Supply 105
Day 49: Firm Foundation 107
Day 50: Cut Yourself Some Slack 111
Day 51: Comparison Trap 113
Day 52: The Measuring Stick 115
Day 53: Workmanship 117
Day 54: Expand My Horizon 119
Day 55: The Hand of God 121
Day 56: Be Bold, Be Adventurous 123
Day 57: The Bitterness Backpack 125
Day 58: The Diving Board 127
Day 59: The Crosswalk 131
Day 60: Enjoy the Journey 133
Works Cited 135
Index 137

INTRODUCTION

August 16, 2020 was an incredibly emotional, confusing day. It was the day I announced to the church, which God allowed me to start and pastor for three years, that I was stepping down from being the pastor. The reason being that I needed healing for my mental health and desperately needed to learn how to better manage it. The weight of pastoring during a pandemic, being a husband, and a father to little ones, while having mental illness, became too heavy. The toll became too great. I knew there was no other option. I couldn't continue leading the church and be a healthy me. But that made the transition no easier. I had, and still have, a deep love for that group of believers. I had poured all of my energy, passion, sweat, and heart into the church for over three years and then one day, I was stepping away from it all...with no game plan or direction for what was next.

As someone who needs structure, I was walking into extremely scary waters. One of the biggest questions I received was what my next step, chapter, job would be. And for the first time in my life, I had NO idea. My answer was simply, *"All I know at this time is that God wants to work on me and provide some sort of healing."* Those next weeks and months were extremely difficult for me. It required me to stop the hustle, the planning, the relying on my power, and to sit in the quietness and ask God to speak. I didn't ask for answers, or a roadmap for the rest of the journey, or even clarity on the next step. I simply prayed, *"God speak to me in the here and now. Help me to see the Jared You see."* In those raw, quiet, ordinary moments, God spoke louder to me than I had ever heard. At times, it felt like He was physically sitting next to me. What He is teaching me in this difficult, but precious season and lessons He helped me understand about past seasons, are all in this devotional book. This 60-day journey is my heart poured out...the bright spots, the low valleys, and most importantly, the God-moments.

It really wasn't until recent years that my eyes have been open to how mental illness is affecting so many others. Mental illness hinders people everywhere from living the quality of life they hope for and even prevents the ability to function in certain capacities. That is why I felt such a strong urge to start a podcast on the subject and write this book. There is no denying that it's not a popular move to share your struggle of mental illness. Although our society and churches, as a whole, have taken a step forward in this regard, there remains a stigma. It is still a taboo topic, which is a sad reality, based off of the number of people who live with a mental illness. It's time for that to change. It's time for us to stand up and say, *"Mental illness is real and normal."* If we want to keep learning how to best manage our mental health, we can't stop until it is viewed in the same way as any other physical disease or deficiency.

My goal in this devotional book is to help equip you and encourage you for the journey of life with mental illness. The aim is not for you to simply get through life, but for you to live fully and love freely with mental illness. I believe that is 100% possible in your life. The number one question I have for you is: For the next 60 days, are you willing to approach our time together with an open heart and mind for what God wants to reveal to you, encourage you with, or teach you? My prayer and hope are that your answer is *"Yes!"*

DAY 1: ONE IS THE LONELIEST NUMBER

GOD'S WORD:

Never will I leave you; never will I forsake you.
Hebrews 13:5

TODAY'S THOUGHT:

I don't know the number of times I have walked into a crowded room and thought, *"No one in here has any idea of what I am battling inside and the hurt I am experiencing."* Have you ever had that thought? Have you walked into a room and felt all alone? That can be the most isolating feeling in the world.

If you broke your foot, the doctor would require you to wear a cast, so that it could heal properly. It would be a physical sign to others that you are in pain and currently limited from some activities. Unfortunately, when you are in need of mental healing, you don't wear a bandage on your head. There is not a visible reminder that you are hurting, in need of healing, and may be limited in certain aspects. As a result, even people who are aware of the battles you are fighting, may not remember in the moment. Regardless if it is intentional or not, this can leave you feeling alone. Isolated. Misunderstood.

In moments like these, try your very best to remember that you are not alone. You have more people in your corner with boxing gloves on, ready to help fight your battles with you, than you may realize. Also, people around you are walking down a similar path as you, and you two have just not crossed paths yet. Most importantly, Hebrews 13:5 assures you that God is always with you. Even if you tried, you could not get away from Him. He has committed to not leave your side. You have the Creator of the universe right there with you. Take comfort in that truth!

QUESTIONS TO CONSIDER:

- Since you don't wear a bandage on your head, are there people in your life that you need to help explain what you are going through, feeling, and experiencing, so that they can better understand you? Who is one person you can tell? Will you commit to having that conversation?

- Does it bring comfort knowing God is always with you? In what ways?

TAKEAWAY:

Make Hebrews 13:5 a daily reminder for yourself. That could look a number of ways:

- Write it out on your bathroom mirror with a dry erase marker.

- Set it as the screensaver on your phone or laptop.

- Write it out on an index card and place it next to your bed or in your car so you see it regularly.

DAY 2: BARELY REACHING FOR COFFEE

GOD'S WORD:

The LORD is near to all who call on him, to all who call on him in truth.
Psalms 145:18

TODAY'S THOUGHT:

Some days (okay, if truth be told...almost EVERY day) the alarm rings, the kids call out or scream at the top of their lungs, the demands of the day are already stacking up, and the only thought that seems to exist is, *"I don't know if I will survive today. I am not sure I have the strength to even turn on the coffee maker."* I refer to this as the *"freight train"* mornings. That term is reserved for the mornings that feel like a freight train ran over your body multiple times during the night. In my household, I think I use the term more days than not.

Let's be honest, when the mornings begin in this way, the day feels like a daunting, uphill battle. The day feels like it can only get worse. You almost just want to get back in bed and try again the next day. But this mindset, as powerful as it may seem, doesn't have to gain control. Before your mind latches onto that perspective and wraps itself around it, stop what you are doing, go to God in prayer, and *"ask for an extra dose of strength from God."* Allow the Giver of life to be your source of nourishment and your supplier of strength.

You don't have to question if God will be receptive to your requests. Scripture makes it clear that when you seek God with a sincere heart, He pulls you close and, in a sense, *"wraps His arms around you."* He longs to hold you and give you everything you need. Keep the line of communication open. Continue to seek the strength of God throughout the day. There is no limit to the amount of strength God is willing to pour into you.

QUESTIONS TO CONSIDER:

- What is your initial response when you start the morning poorly...convince yourself the day will only get worse or seek the strength of God?

- In a typical week, what other times of the day do you need to call on God to provide an extra dose of strength?

TAKEAWAY:

It helps to have a memorable phrase already picked out that you can pray to God as often as you need throughout the day. It will help re-center your mind and attention to help take the pressure off. For example, one prayer I have used before is simply, *God, give me what I need today.*

DAY 3: WHERE IS THE LOVE?

GOD'S WORD:

See what great love the Father has lavished on us, that we should be called
children of God! And that is what we are! The reason the world does not
know us is that it did not know him.

1 John 3:1

TODAY'S THOUGHT:

Today when you woke up, you may have felt that you don't measure
up in some way; that you fall short of certain standards that limit
you from truly being loved. If so, you are definitely not alone in that
feeling. Because of today's culture, it's rather easy to fall into this way
of thinking. Society has set a standard for what is worthy and what is
valuable, and that standard is in opposition to what God says. Society
claims you are valuable if you succeed in your career by making
more money than you did the year before. Getting a bigger office.
Making better grades than everyone else in your class. Buying a huge
house. Having thousands upon thousands of social media followers.
Once you start living to reach this standard, your identity becomes
intertwined with this mindset. That is a scary reality, because what
happens when life doesn't go quite as planned? You are left feeling
like a failure. Feeling like you have nothing and are nothing.

This isn't the easiest devotional for me to write, because I know
the feeling too well. I placed a big portion of my identity in pastoring
a church and what I viewed as success within that role. When I
stepped down from pastoring, the transition was extremely difficult.
Who was I now? What was my purpose? Thank God, in my time of

healing, a friend of mine named Stephen, reminded me of a truth I desperately needed to hear. This was the text he sent me:

> *Thinking of you this morning man. You're a loved son, Jared. Always have been, always will be. Fully loved, fully accepted, fully affirmed in Him. You've gotten the thumbs up from the only thumb that matters.*

No matter how you feel right now, *you are a loved son or daughter.* No matter how you perceive life to be going, *you are a loved son or daughter.* Whether you are on a mountaintop or in the valley during a period of healing, *you are a loved son or daughter.*

This statement is the most important truth for you and about you. There is nothing you could do or not do to change that. God doesn't love you any less when life goes differently than you planned. That takes the pressure away from performance. Being loved by Christ makes you more valuable than anything else this world could offer you. Dwell on that truth every single morning and let it dictate your perspective that day. Because like Stephen said: *You've gotten the thumbs up from the only thumb that matters.*

Questions To Consider:

- Whose approval have you been chasing after that you need to let go of?
- If you truly believed this truth, how would it change your perspective?

Takeaway:

Say this prayer: *God, I want to focus on Your love for me. My identity is in You and I have approval from the One that matters. I will rest in that truth today. Amen.*

DAY 4: IT'S OKAY TO NOT BE OKAY

GOD'S WORD:

But we have this treasure in jars of clay to show that this all-surpassing power is from God and not from us. We are hard pressed on every side, but not crushed; perplexed, but not in despair; persecuted, but not abandoned; struck down, but not destroyed. We always carry around in our body the death of Jesus, so that the life of Jesus may also be revealed in our body. For we who are alive are always being given over to death for Jesus' sake, so that his life may also be revealed in our mortal body. So then, death is at work in us, but life is at work in you.

2 Corinthians 4:7–12

TODAY'S THOUGHT:

My counselor recently called me out on something. Every time she would ask how I was doing in the beginning of the conversation, I would automatically answer with, *"I'm doing good; thank you for asking."* And then the rest of the counseling session would show that I was, in fact, not okay. Why is it that we feel pressured to not admit that, at the moment, we are struggling? Why is it that we believe if we share what we are going through or the current state we are in, we have to make it seem like it's not really a struggle anymore and we are in a better place? That's not real. It's not healthy. It's not okay. Of course, we want to make healthy progress at the right pace, but there is a proper time to not be okay and for that to be acceptable. Thinking you have to move to a state of complete well-being immediately is not realistic and does not end pretty. You end up only masking how you really feel and not reaching out for help or healing.

One of the most freeing aspects for me occurred in one of the first episodes of my podcast when I admitted that I was still in the middle of my brokenness. I explained that I had resources around me to help me move forward. I was heading in the right direction to find healing. I was looking toward better days, but I wasn't there yet. I plain out admitted that I wasn't okay. I was nervous about sharing that, but once I did, I felt a weight released off of my shoulders.

It's okay to not be okay, as long as you know which direction you are headed. The broken times can actually lead to powerful moments in your life and the lives of others. Warren Wiersbe explained it as, *"Sometimes God permits our vessels to be jarred so that some of the treasure will spill out and enrich others."* The treasure Warren Wiersbe is referring to is God and His love. Being real and authentic about the fact that you are in the middle of your weakness, allows God to shine even brighter. It draws people to you and allows opportunities for "God conversations." Trust me; it's okay to not be okay.

QUESTIONS TO CONSIDER:

- Do you struggle with admitting that you are not okay? What reasons prevent you from doing so?

- What difference would it make in your life to be okay with not being okay?

- What kind of conversations might come about from your authenticity?

TAKEAWAY:

Say this prayer: God, use my time of weakness. Use my brokenness to draw me and others close to You. Thank You for Your faithfulness and love for me. Amen.

---

[1]Warren Wiersbe, *The Wiersbe Bible Commentary*, NT (Colorado Springs: David C. Cook, 2007), 513.

DAY 5: LET GO OF EMBARRASSMENT

GOD'S WORD:

Not that I have already obtained all this, or have already arrived at my goal, but I press on to take hold of that for which Christ Jesus took hold of me.

Philippians 3:12

TODAY'S THOUGHT:

One of the most common things that I hear on my podcast and in conversations with others is the struggle of feeling embarrassed about mental illness. Mental illness is difficult to describe. You can't see it. You don't know if anyone else is dealing with this struggle like you are. Even though the mental illness is causing real pain, sometimes it feels easier to bottle it up and not say anything to anyone. One of the main causes is embarrassment.

For me, growing up in church, I was embarrassed because I equated my mental illness with not having enough faith in God or that I wasn't trusting Him enough with my life. I thought, *"Well, maybe if I pray harder or try to believe more, this monster in my mind will leave."* I felt like I couldn't tell anyone, because I was surrounded by numerous other Christians. What would they think? How would they respond? So, I pushed through for as long as I could, hoping it would go away. I allowed my embarrassment to keep me from much needed support. Hiding behind my embarrassment brought along a lot of pain.

If there is anything that I want you to focus on today, it's this: You don't need to feel embarrassed about mental illness. You're not crazy in the mind. It doesn't mean you don't have enough faith in

God. It doesn't mean you are weak. It's a real issue, just like a broken bone is. Every single person is struggling with some type of battle; yours just happens to be mental illness. The sooner you can let go of the feeling of embarrassment, the more freeing it will become for you. Don't allow embarrassment to keep you from the help and support you deserve. Let go of the embarrassment, it doesn't belong any longer.

QUESTIONS TO CONSIDER:

- Have you been embarrassed of your mental illness? If you were to examine it, what would be the core reason?

- If the feelings of embarrassment were no longer there, who would you tell? What resource would you reach out for?

TAKEAWAY:

Say this prayer: Lord, I want to view my mental illness for what it is and seek support with it. Help me find my security and identity in You. Amen.

DAY 6: COUNTING SHEEP

In peace I will lie down and sleep,
for you alone, Lord, make me dwell in safety.

Psalms 4:8

TODAY'S THOUGHT:

Have you ever run out of gas while driving? Some people pull over to a gas station as soon as the light pops up and the ding noise indicates low gas. Others like to put it off, and off, and off, until they run completely out of gas and are stuck looking for people to help push the vehicle. Unless you have made the switch to electric cars, your car can't function without gas in the tank. If you run out of gas, you can't just get out and rub the hood of your vehicle and say nice things to your car until it gets motivated and keeps driving. This isn't the movie *Transformers.*[2] It doesn't work like that. Unfortunately, this can be the mindset when it comes to mental, physical, and emotional health. Picture those three as tanks. You only have a certain amount of gas in your tanks each day. If you run out, you aren't able to function. You can't just push through it and hope for the best. That's not the way it works. To stay within your capacity level, you need proper rest. Without it, you will be running on empty, which leads to restlessness and eventually breaking down.

For the next few days, when you read the word *"rest,"* think of it in terms of being replenished. It's the thought of being filled up or built

---

[2]John Rogers, Roberto Orci and Alex Kurtzman, *Transformers* (2007; North America: DreamWorks Pictures.)

up again. This will apply to mental, physical, and emotional health. One of the best ways to make sure you are being replenished, especially with mental illness, is to create and maintain healthy rhythms. A rhythm is *"a strong, regular, repeated pattern."* Much of God's creation, if not every part, was established with some type of rhythm. The rhythm of day and night: light and darkness. The rhythm of the ocean tide: the tide comes in, the tide goes out. The rhythm of breathing: you breathe in, you breathe out. Even while you sleep, your lungs take in oxygen and release it.

Today, let's focus on physical rest, with the main component being your sleep schedule. Because what do you do every night before you get up and start the day? Sleep. Making sure your day begins successfully, actually starts the night before with getting the right amount of sleep. The quality of your sleep dictates your energy level the next day. The National Sleep Foundation guidelines advise that adults need 7-9 hours of sleep and teenagers need 8-10 hours of sleep.[3] You may say, *"Well, I can operate on a lot less than that."* That may be true, but it doesn't mean that you wouldn't be healthier and more effective with more sleep. Studies show that some of the effects of getting less sleep than your body needs are fatigue, lack of motivation, moodiness, increased risk of depression, inability to cope with stress, and difficulty managing emotions.[4] That is a big deal and can play a massive role in decreased mental health.

Sadly, one's sleep schedule is rarely protected. This is something you can control starting today. Don't sacrifice sleep for things of little to no value. Make sleep a priority. Give yourself the best opportunity to not only create healthy rhythms, but to maintain them.

QUESTIONS TO CONSIDER:

- Do you have a healthy sleep schedule rhythm? Approximately how many hours do you typically sleep?

---

[3] Melinda Smith, M.A., Lawrence Robinson, and Robert Segal, M.A., "Sleep Needs," *Help Guide*, last modified October 2020,
https://www.helpguide.org/articles/sleep/sleep-needs-get-the-sleep-you-need.htm
[4] Ibid.

- What do you need to do during the evening to make sure that you get to bed at a good time?

TAKEAWAY:

Studies show that looking at screens right before you go to bed stimulates your brain. Try not getting on your phone, laptop, or watching TV at least an hour before you lay down.

Don't sacrifice sleep for things of little to no value.

DAY 7: START THE DAY RIGHT

GOD'S WORD:

In the early morning, while it was still dark, Jesus got up, left the house, and went away to a secluded place, and was praying there.

Mark 1:35

TODAY'S THOUGHT:

Another rhythm you can create or tweak, to make sure you are being replenished daily, is your morning routine. When battling mental illness, finding ways to achieve early wins in the day makes a huge difference. You want to start off on the right foot. Starting your day rushed, unable to find what you need, forgetting to put on deodorant, leads to more anxiety and stress (and a loss of friends from the odor). Then you are starting the workday, school day, or time with the kids at home on a bad note. An Olympic runner would never start a race without already having tied their shoes, stretched, and prepared themselves mentally. Otherwise, they can plan on a sluggish start to the race or a pulled muscle. Each day of your life is a part of the race and how you start each lap matters.

If you create a healthy sleep rhythm, like we discussed yesterday, then it is easier to establish a healthy morning routine rhythm. For me, that routine includes waking up with enough time before the family wakes up to do my quiet time, drink a cup of coffee (or two or three), and then exercise for at least 30 minutes. Before the responsibilities of the day begin, I've already achieved three wins, which create a positive feeling about the day. Those mornings are much more effective than when I choose to get off of my rhythm. Not only that, but they are wins that improve my life. Exercising improves my physical health and mental health and time with God is the best medicine for my soul.

Establish a morning routine that prepares your mind, body, and soul for the day. Follow the example of Jesus by spending time with God before anything else. Start the day with some early wins!

QUESTIONS TO CONSIDER:

- What does your morning routine currently look like? Are you following the example of Jesus?

- Do you need to get up at an earlier time than you currently are?

- Are there wins you can add to your morning that will increase your optimism for the day? If so, what are they?

TAKEAWAY:

Try to prepare as much as you can the night before. Pick out your exercise clothes, gather your bible, notebook, and pen, and prepare your coffee, so that you only have to hit the brew button. This will help eliminate anxiety and the need to scramble in the morning, as well as give your excuses less leverage.

DAY 8: BENEFITS OF EXERCISE

God's Word:

*Beloved, I pray that all may go well with you and that you may be in good
health, as it goes well with your soul.*

3 John 1:2

Today's Thought:

When you are in a low mental state, the last thing you may want
to do is exercise. That sounds like torture when your tank is on
empty. Honestly, eating nails can sound more appealing than moving
around when you are in a low place. Often times, exercise is pushed
aside for a matter of time, which is unfortunate because it positively
affects your mental health. The reason it is so beneficial is because
God created your body in a way that exercise releases chemicals like
endorphins and serotonin in your brain that can enhance your sense
of well-being. It can also improve your sleep, which we, in prior days,
discussed the importance of.

When you hear the word *"exercise,"* you may automatically think
of sprinting laps around a track or moving around non-stop in Cross-
Fit. While it can be those, exercise is simply planned physical activity
that works your muscles. That can range from washing your car,
gardening, walking around the block, to running, bike riding, playing sports, lifting weights. You simply pick something that requires
energy on your part and then create a steady rhythm.

The Mayo Clinic recommends 30 minutes or more of exercise for
three to five days a week. When you think about it, 30 minutes is a
tiny sliver of time in comparison to the whole day. Whether it's in

the morning, during your lunch break, in the evening, or broken up between those times, make it a regular part of your week. View it as a medication that improves your mental health and physical health. There are too many benefits to not make it a weekly rhythm.

QUESTIONS TO CONSIDER:

- 1 Corinthians 6:19 says that "your body is a temple" from God. Are you taking care of the body God has entrusted you with?
- What type of physical activity would be best for you to start this week?
- Who can you share your goal of exercising with that can keep you accountable?

TAKEAWAY:

If you don't already know, you will quickly figure out if you prefer exercising alone or with a partner/group. I prefer to put headphones on and exercise alone, but many people I know would despise exercising in isolation. If that is you, find a workout partner ASAP. Don't let that deter your progress.

DAY 9: BRAIN FUEL

GOD'S WORD:

> *So whether you eat or drink or whatever you do,*
> *do it all for the glory of God.*
> 1 Corinthians 10:31

TODAY'S THOUGHT:

For the longest time, I knew the correlation of my diet with my physical health, but it took a while for me to connect what I ate with my mental health. As I did some research, I was blown away by the degree that mental health is affected by what is put into the body. I am NO expert in this field, so I will leave it to the professionals to explain. Dr. Eva Selhub, with the *Harvard Health Blog*, explains:

> *Your brain requires a constant supply of fuel. That "fuel" comes from the foods you eat — and what's in that fuel makes all the difference. Put simply, what you eat directly affects the structure and function of your brain and, ultimately, your mood...Eating high-quality foods that contain lots of vitamins, minerals, and antioxidants nourishes the brain and protects it from oxidative stress — the "waste" (free radicals) produced when the body uses oxygen, which can damage cells.*[5]

We wouldn't be surprised if our cars didn't function well after we filled it up with low quality or watered-down fuel. But at times, we

---

[5]Ibid.

don't think twice about the fuel we pump into our bodies and how it will affect the brain. Dr. Selhub also explained that a diet that includes a high volume of refined sugars has been linked with impaired brain function and worsening mood disorders, such as depression.[6]

For you, getting to the type of healthy diet you want may take time and that's okay. This isn't a sprint; it's a marathon. Start taking steps to make changes to improve the quality of your brain's fuel. The good news is that this is an area you do have control over. How you decide to handle this area will either set you up for success or worsen your mental illness. Ultimately, you can bring glory to God by taking care of the body He gave you. Let's begin moving in the right direction!

QUESTIONS TO CONSIDER:

- How can being mindful of what you eat bring glory to God?

- What is one thing you could tweak, add, or take out of your diet this week that would improve your brain's fuel?

- Is there someone you need to reach out to for accountability? Who?

TAKEAWAY:

There are numerous resources for healthy eating habits. Try googling the type of diet or meal plan you are looking for and favorite a website you think you would like to try out. It is all about taking small steps.

---

[6]Ibid.

DAY 10: THE PACE OF LIFE

God's Word:

The apostles gathered around Jesus and reported to him all they had done and taught. Then, because so many people were coming and going that they did not even have a chance to eat, he said to them, "Come with me by yourselves to a quiet place and get some rest."

Mark 6:30–31

Today's Thought:

The "American Dream" of success, money, power, recognition can be incredibly enticing. Everyone is told that it is within reach if you only work hard enough. The idea is if you want to *be* more, you have to *do* more. You have to sleep less. You have to go, go, go to move closer to the goal. That leads to non-stop thinking of what needs to be done, done better, or how to do even more. Any extra moments in the day are filled with more activities, more projects, more goals. You are left with zero bandwidth to simply rest and to enjoy what God has created and what God is doing all around you.

Where does that leave us, especially those with mental illness? It leads to being worn down, running on fumes, becoming a shell of yourself, and feeling less than others. That is not how God designed the world to function. That is not how He designed you to live your life. Let me throw a crazy proposition out to you...maybe the thing that would lead to the most success for you this week is to do less. You probably never thought you would aim to do less, in order to accomplish more in life, but that's the goal. It's fine to not keep up with what others seem to be achieving on social media, or at work, or at the local park.

One of the healthiest steps I took was convincing myself it was okay to slow down. I had to learn to live *with* my mental illness and not pretend it wasn't there. That automatically made a difference when I made decisions on how much I would or would not participate in during the week. It wasn't healthy for me to push myself to the point of running on fumes. It is never good for you or the people around you, if you hit a wall by overcommitting yourself.

You don't need to feel bad about going against the grain and slowing down to a healthy pace. Sure, not everyone will understand, but that's not what is most important...your health is. Don't ever apologize for taking care of yourself.

Questions To Consider:

- What type of refreshing activity can you do to re-energize yourself when you take time to rest this week?

- Will you commit to find time for it at least once this week? What day?

Takeaway:

Say this prayer: God, I know I need to slow down and find rest. I will choose to find my rest in You. Help me see what You are doing in and around me. Amen.

DAY 11: THE GREATEST DECISION

God's Word:

If you declare with your mouth, "Jesus is Lord," and believe in your heart that God raised him from the dead, you will be saved. For it is with your heart that you believe and are justified, and it is with your mouth that you profess your faith and are saved.

Romans 10:9–10

Today's Thought:

Have you been going through life, feeling like you are missing something? You get through each week and say, *"There's got to be more. There has to be a bigger purpose."* Every person feels this at some point in life. People try to fill that hole with career success, a big house, social media following, parenting, excelling in sports or school. These can bring happiness for a moment, but fade quickly, leaving you where you started. I truly believe that the purpose you are looking for is found in Jesus. My purpose in life is completely centered on my relationship with God. Everything else stems off of that foundation.

We were created by God to have a relationship with Him. But something happens the moment we are born into a fallen world. *"For all have sinned and fall short of the glory of God."* (Romans 3:23) We all sin. We do things we are not proud of. We say hurtful things. There are consequences for our wrongdoings. *"For the wages of sin is death, but the gift of God is eternal life in Christ Jesus our Lord."* (Romans 6:23) The consequence for sin is death; eternal separation from God.

Unless those sins are dealt with, we are all destined for hell. The penalty will be held against us and nothing in our power can fix the broken relationship. *"But God demonstrates his own love for us in this:*

While we were still sinners, Christ died for us." (Romans 5:8) God sent His only Son, Jesus, to take your place, to be your substitute. Jesus took on your sin, your junk, your mess. He took it all to the cross, because it had to be dealt with. Jesus died on the cross, so you would not have to. He did not stay dead, though. He rose again, so that your sins could be forgiven. He rose, so you could have true life here on earth and eternal life with Him in heaven.

God offers the free gift of salvation to all who call upon Him, knowing Jesus died and rose from the dead, asking for forgiveness of sins and for Christ to come into their lives. The greatest decision I ever made was accepting Jesus as my Lord and Savior. I cannot imagine trying to battle mental illness without God. Is today the day you make that decision for yourself?

Questions To Consider:

- Have you asked Jesus to come into your life and forgive you of your sins? Are you ready to make that decision today?

- If you have made that decision, who in your life do you need to share these truths with?

Takeaway:

If you have never asked Jesus into your life and would like to, you can ask Him right now. Say this prayer: *God, I know I have sinned. Please forgive me. I confess with my mouth and believe with my heart that Jesus died on the cross for my sins and rose from the dead. Come into my life and be my Lord and Savior. Thank you for forgiving me and saving me. Amen!*

DAY 12: BURDENS OF THE DAY

GOD'S WORD:

*Come to me, all you who are weary and burdened, and I will give you rest.
Take my yoke upon you and learn from me, for I am gentle and humble in
heart, and you will find rest for your souls. For my yoke is easy and my
burden is light.*
Matthew 11:28–30

TODAY'S THOUGHT:

In biblical times, yokes were used by farmers to link oxen together.
The yoke was then attached to a plow. Both oxen would work together,
pulling the plow. The farmers didn't just randomly pick which oxen
would be paired together. They would often take a young ox and
partner him with a mature, experienced ox that was stronger. The
stronger ox would lead the way, set the speed, and pull most of the
weight. The young ox had one job and that was to follow the direction
and speed that was set for them by the mature ox. As long as the
young ox didn't try to take control, go a different direction, or change
the pace, everything would work smoothly. The mature ox would
carry most of the load and set a sustainable pace, until the work was
completed.

This makes what Matthew says in chapter 11 a life-changing
opportunity. You are that young ox, who has a field of life in front
of you. Not only is this life difficult to walk through, not only is the
work draining, not only are you straining to pull the plow, the burden,
for the day, but you are doing all of this while living with a mental
illness. It can feel impossible.

Knowing that would be the case, Jesus calls you, while you are weary and burdened, to come to Him to find rest for your souls. Jesus wants you to yoke yourself to Him, the "mature ox," so that you can walk together. He wants to lead the way, set the pace, set the direction, and carry most of the weight. He wants you to simply follow His lead and the pace that He sets. Don't let pride or a sense of unworthiness lead you into pulling the plow for the day by yourself. Lean into Christ today. Go to Him and allow Him to help carry your burden.

QUESTIONS TO CONSIDER:

- Do you tend to try and carry the burdens of the day by yourself? Why or why not?
- What specific burdens have you been carrying for too long?
- What hinders you from bringing those to the feet of Jesus?

TAKEAWAY:

Say this prayer: Lord, I am weary and burdened. I choose to come to You, knowing You will give true rest for my soul. Help me to remember that I don't have to bear my burdens alone. Amen.

DAY 13: CHAINS

GOD'S WORD:

*Now I want you to know, brothers and sisters, that what has happened to
me has actually served to advance the gospel. As a result, it has become
clear throughout the whole palace guard and to everyone else that I am in
chains for Christ. And because of my chains, most of the brothers and
sisters have become confident in the Lord and dare all the more to proclaim
the gospel without fear.*
Philippians 1:12–14

TODAY'S THOUGHT:

For years, I viewed my depression and anxiety as *chains. Limitations.
Handicaps. Hopeless barriers.* I had passions and visions of ways I
could help lead people to Christ, but there was always a little voice
in my head that said, *"Don't get too excited, Jared. Remember you deal
with mental illness."* Can you relate? When you think about helping
other people or making a difference for God, the idea may sound
good, but the practical aspects of it get fuzzy. Maybe you have had
thoughts similar to mine: *"With my mental illness, I am limited in
what I can do, unlike someone who does not have these struggles. I don't
have the energy, the capacity, consistency to do anything that matters."*

A few years back, I was leading a study through the book of
Philippians in the New Testament, when God started to change my
perspective on this. As Paul, the author of Philippians, was preaching
the gospel of Jesus Christ, he was arrested and put in the Roman
prison system. I'm sure, at first, he had similar thoughts and felt
defeated that his plans were put on hold. He felt God leading him
to preach, but now he had chains around his limbs, limiting him

from doing what he set out to do. But then God started to reveal to Paul opportunities to advance the gospel right where he was, that wouldn't have been available to Paul otherwise. Paul's chains granted him exposure to some powerful people in the Roman government. As a prisoner, his case was taken to the officials in Caesar's court, where he boldly proclaimed the truth. He began to tell the Roman soldiers and other prisoners about Jesus. Paul's chains advanced the gospel in a way that he would have never imagined.

My question for you is this: what if your chains are exactly what is needed to accomplish God's purposes at this moment? What if your chains of mental illness actually held greater potential for good than you could have ever thought? Sometimes the things that we so desperately desire to get rid of, are actually the greatest tools we have to offer God in that season. You may be able to help someone else walk through a similar struggle you have, that you wouldn't have been able to help otherwise. God has you right where you need to be, and your chains aren't dealbreakers.

QUESTIONS TO CONSIDER:

- Think back on your life...what opportunities have you had because of your chains?

- Who is one person that God is bringing to mind that deals with something similar to you that you can encourage?

TAKEAWAY:

Say this prayer: Lord, help me view my chains in a way that I never have before. Open my eyes to the opportunities You have placed all around me. I want to glorify You during this time. Amen.

DAY 14: WHERE CAN I TURN?

GOD'S WORD:

*Where there is no guidance, a people falls, but in an abundance of
counselors there is safety.*

Proverbs 11:14

TODAY'S THOUGHT:

After my panic attack and after stepping away from pastoring, I
knew I needed help. I needed resources and aid. The pride in me
wanted to figure everything out alone, but God helped me realize the
foolishness in that flawed thinking. I had pastored for years, and even
though it was not professional counseling, I had offered counseling
to individuals, couples, and families numerous times. Because of that,
I convinced myself that participating in counseling myself wouldn't
be beneficial.

It took godly people in my life that kept nudging me in the right
direction, until I finally called and set up a counseling session with a
Christian counselor. Let me tell you...it was one of the best decisions
of my life. Beforehand, I couldn't have comprehended the healing and
insight I would receive through it. It was not my counselor telling
me what I was doing wrong and how I should live. But instead, my
counselor asked the right questions so that I was able to figure that
out, as God spoke to me. I truly believe I would be nowhere near as
healthy without that resource of counseling.

I share all of that because you or someone you love might be
right where I was prior to counseling; unsure of the value, tainted
perspective, not willing to admit you need help in that way. As you
take a look inside, if you find any speck of truth in those statements,

counseling might be a wonderful resource for you. Maybe you've tried before in the past and it felt ineffective and a waste of time. I encourage you to give it one more try. Counseling does require the right fit between you and a counselor. Your personality simply may have not clicked with your prior counselor. That is okay. But it shouldn't stop you from trying again.

Remember: counseling doesn't make you weaker, less of a person, or crazy. It makes you wise and strong for wanting to be the healthiest you.

QUESTIONS TO CONSIDER:

- Do you think some type of counseling would be beneficial for you? What has held you back from wanting to pursue or stick with counseling?
- Do you know someone that counseling might benefit?

TAKEAWAY:

If the answer is 'yes,' let today be the day you take a step forward.

- If it is for you, simply call a counseling center, ask for more information and any other questions you have. (I recommend a Christian counseling center, because they will approach it from a biblical perspective.)
- If it is for someone else, commit to pray for them. If God gives you a peace, talk to them about counseling. Even if they are resistant at first, God will use your kind act in some way.

DAY 15: YOUR SOUL NEEDS WORSHIP

GOD'S WORD:

Because your love is better than life, my lips will glorify you. I will praise
you as long as I live, and in your name I will lift up my hands. Because
you are my help, I sing in the shadow of your wings. I cling to you; your
right hand upholds me.

Psalms 63:3-8

TODAY'S THOUGHT:

This verse gives me goosebumps every time I read it. My mind
automatically goes to the times that I have experienced intimate, deep
worship. During these instances, I was telling God how marvelous,
how captivating, how amazing He is. I was singing songs of praises
and my lips weren't the only part of my body that was participating.
My body was swaying, my hands were raised up as high as they
could go. I wasn't thinking about anyone or anything, other than my
Savior, and it was beautiful. It was exactly what my soul needed.

You were created to worship God. Your soul longs for it. It
desperately needs it. Your mental health feels refreshed during and
after truly worshipping God. Worshipping God is not some type
of cheat code to help mental health. Worshipping God is how you
were designed to live, so, of course, it would enhance every aspect of
your life, mental health included. When you truly contemplate what
Jesus did on the cross for you; how He died in your place, but then
rose from the dead three days later, you can't help but worship God.
When you reflect on all of the wonderful gifts that God has blessed
you with, you can't help but lift the name of God on high. When you

think back to all of the times God led you through a difficult time, you can't help but surrender yourself in worship.

Whether you are at church, listening to the radio in the car, watching a worship set on YouTube, at home with your guitar, or singing in the shower, forget about everything else in the moment and sing the lyrics to that worship song with, not only your lips, but also your heart. Your soul needs it.

QUESTIONS TO CONSIDER:

- Does worshipping God in song come easy to you?

- Are there opportunities every week for you to worship? If not, what can you do to make sure those opportunities are there?

TAKEAWAY:

I don't listen to only worship music, but I have been aiming to listen to it more, because of the importance of having the lyrics soak into my mind. I decided I wanted to add it into my week on a more regular basis by listening to worship music during certain workouts I do every week. Is there a time that you could incorporate worship music into your week (driving, doing dishes, exercising, folding laundry, walking)?

DAY 16: HOPE FOR THE HOPELESS

GOD'S WORD:

But those who hope in the LORD will renew their strength. They will soar on wings like eagles; they will run and not grow weary, they will walk and not be faint.

Isaiah 40:31

TODAY'S THOUGHT:

If I had to sum up in one word the state that I was in the day after my panic attack, I would use the word *"HOPELESS."* Just the day before, my anxiety had risen to a level that I had never experienced before, sending me into a state where I lost all control and had a panic attack. In the dark days that followed, I couldn't help but wonder if I would ever be able to live my life again, at least how I had prior to this. I didn't know if I would be able to be the father and husband that I felt my family needed, or manage my anxiety while working a job, or find any type of joy in life again. My hope tank was completely on empty.

Have you had days, weeks, or periods of time where you experienced the same type of feelings? Times where your hope had been ripped away and you couldn't even find a glimmer of hope in the distance? Maybe you are right in the middle of hopelessness right now. If so, my heart goes out to you.

The journey for me since that dark, hopeless season has had its fair share of lightbulb moments and *"face on the ground crying"* periods. But the number one truth that rings louder than anything is that my hope is not found in me, my accomplishments, or my ability to manage my mental health. My hope is in the Lord. He is the One that provides the air under my wings, who picks me up when I fall, who provides strength each and every day.

The same is 100% true for you, as well. No matter how crippling your mental illness may seem. No matter if you are standing tall or with your face down in the dirt. No matter what others say or do...your hope does not come from you. It does not come from others. It does not come from this world. Your hope comes from the Lord. That hope is not affected by your circumstances. Hope from God is ALWAYS available to you. Sit and rest in that hope today.

Questions To Consider:

- Where, what, or in who do you tend to look to for hope?

- Has that source of hope let you down at any point? How so?

- Will you make God your source of strength and hope?

Takeaway:

Say this prayer: Lord, the burden of life can feel so heavy at times. I do not want to buckle under the pressure and start to believe my hope is being stripped away. My hope is found in You and You alone. Thank You for providing hope in my life. Amen.

DAY 17: WHEN ANXIETY ATTACKS

GOD'S WORD:

Cast all your anxiety on him because he cares for you.
1 Peter 5:7

TODAY'S THOUGHT:

Before most arcades switched to electronic tickets, there was a vivid image throughout the entire arcade. The image included children, with smiles on their faces, running to the next arcade game they wanted to play. No objects in their hands. No worries on their minds. A few steps behind them, was the parent trying to keep up with their child, with game tickets in their hands, pockets, and between their toes. The children would win the tickets and instead of carrying them everywhere they went, they would immediately *cast* the tickets onto the parents. In doing so, they didn't have to carry or worry about them anymore. The parent did both of those for them.

In a similar way, God is willing to carry your anxieties for you. He tells you to bring them to Him and let Him carry them for you. If you are anything like me, you deal with anxiety on a regular basis. There are things throughout the whole day that make you anxious. It can feel as if this verse was meant for others but wouldn't apply to you since the anxiety is constant. You can't miss the key word here, though, which is the word *"all."* Not some. Not most. Cast ALL of your anxiety on the Father. God is big enough to handle every single one of your anxieties. Even if it feels like it's every 10 minutes, go to God, and let Him know what is making you anxious. Ask Him to carry the burden for you, and then hand it over like game tickets.

To do so, though, you have to believe the second part of the verse: *because He cares for you.* In your heart, you have to truly believe that God loves you and cares for you in a deeper sense than you could ever comprehend. The more you believe that truth, the easier it becomes to approach God and *cast* your anxieties on Him.

QUESTIONS TO CONSIDER:

- What anxieties do you deal with in your life? Which ones do you need to hand over to God today?

- What is holding you back from doing so? Why do you think that is?

TAKEAWAY:

Try not to be generic about your anxiety when you pray to God. Today, write out specifically what is making you anxious. Then, one by one, cross out each anxiety as you pray "God, I'm handing this to You."

DAY 18: BE STILL AND ALLOW GOD TO BE GOD

GOD'S WORD:

Be still, and know that I am God. I will be exalted among the nations, I will be exalted in the earth!
Psalms 46:10

TODAY'S THOUGHT:

The context of this verse is war. The Israelites were about to be attacked by the Assyrian army. Of course, their natural instinct was to freak out and scramble. But they had the ultimate weapon on their side, something that the Assyrians did not...God. If they would follow God and allow Him to lead, He would protect them. He would defeat the Assyrian army. The Israelites submitted themselves and turned to God and an angel of the Lord came and defeated their enemies. God delivered them, like He had promised. He was their refuge and strength in times of trouble.

Right now, your life may feel like a war zone. There may be many battles that you are currently fighting, one being the battle of mental health. Your tendency may be to try to resolve your situation in your own power and strength. You were never meant to do that. God has promised to be your refuge and strength. He calls you to be still and know that He is God. "Be still," literally means "Take your hands off! Relax!" We like to be in control of our own lives and have a hard time giving the reigns over to God. But God tells us to take our hands off and allow God to be God.

You cannot win this battle on your own, no matter how hard you push and strain. The best action you can take is to stop, even in the midst of the battle, and pray to God. Ask Him to protect and deliver you. This does not mean that you sit back and never do anything to help in the process. You still have to take steps as God leads you. But it is in His timing, based on His plan. Be still and allow God to be God.

QUESTIONS TO CONSIDER:

- Does the thought of being still in the midst of chaos sound realistic for your life? Why or why not?

- When has God provided for you in the past? In what circumstances?

- Do you believe He will protect and deliver you again?

TAKEAWAY:

Say this prayer: Lord, I feel like a battle is raging all around me. I need Your protection and deliverance. I surrender my life to You. I trust You. I choose to be still and know that You are God. Thank You for Your faithfulness. Amen.

DAY 19: CHOOSING LOVE

GOD'S WORD:

Love is patient, love is kind. It does not envy, it does not boast, it is not proud. It does not dishonor others, it is not self-seeking, it is not easily angered, it keeps no record of wrongs. Love does not delight in evil but rejoices with the truth. It always protects, always trusts, always hopes, always perseveres. Love never fails.

1 Corinthians 13:4–8

TODAY'S THOUGHT:

Today is dedicated to those who have someone in their life that battles mental illness (if you have mental illness, please do not check out; today's thought is for you, as well). Mental illness is extremely difficult to understand. It is easy to forget that someone struggles with something you cannot see. At times, as the supporter, it will feel like you are carrying a heavy weight. You may not feel qualified or patient enough to help your loved one in the way he or she needs.

That is where 1 Corinthians 13 comes in. In your flesh, you may not feel like being patient, kind, selfless, and persevering. The key word there is "*feel.*" Yes, you will not always feel like it, but love is not based on feelings. Love is a commitment. An action. A decision to do what is best for the other person. Jesus did not feel like dying on the cross. He chose to do it out of love, because it was best for you and me.

When your loved one says a situation is causing them severe stress, *choose love.* When they tell you that the thought of going out tonight is leaving them anxious, *choose love.* When they are in a low place and have a hard time making decisions, *choose love.* When their mood seems to change drastically, quickly, *choose love*. Decide to show love, even though you do not feel like it. Why? Because, love never fails and love does what is best for the other person.

Those with mental illness, help your loved ones help you. Your supporters are not choosing to forget about your struggles; but at times, it simply does not come to mind. The way you can help with that is to communicate clearly, what it is that you feel and why. Understand that this is an area that will take time to see consistency in; it typically does not happen overnight. But it starts with choosing love today!

Questions To Consider:

- For the supporters: When is it hardest to display patience with your loved one? Is there a common thread?

- Do you feel there is clear communication? If not, would better communication make it easier to be patient?

- Both sides: Will you commit to communicate clearly and early?

Takeaway:

Have a conversation today or sometime this week, with the individual that you support in their battle against mental illness. Explain what God revealed to you as you read today's devotional and assure them that they have your full support.

DAY 20: I NEED ANSWERS

GOD'S WORD:

If any of you lacks wisdom, you should ask God, who gives generously to all without finding fault, and it will be given to you.

James 1:5

TODAY'S THOUGHT:

Decisions, decisions, decisions. Who knows how many countless decisions you make on a regular basis? Those range from what you will eat in the morning, to how many times you will watch the TV show *The Office*,[7] to daily tasks at work or school. What happens when you do too much of anything without a break? You get fatigued. This can actually happen when making long sessions of decisions. This is something called *"decision fatigue."* I was first introduced to the term and explanation of it by my good friend, Billy, who helped provide valuable insight on this topic. Billy runs a company, which means he makes decisions and gives the thumbs up or down, throughout the entire workday. Billy also lives with mental illness. He explained to me that it can get to the place, if he's not careful, where it's difficult to make additional decisions for him and his family, especially big decisions, because of decision fatigue.

Have you ever felt like that? You make minor decisions throughout each day, every day and it slowly wears you down. Out of nowhere, you are suddenly hit with a larger decision that affects more of your life or the life of others, and it stops you in your tracks. You're already fatigued from numerous prior decisions and you battle

---

[7] *The Office*, Deedle-Dee Productions and Reveille Productions, 2005-2013.

mental illness, so you don't know where to even start. In moments like these, it is easy to get overwhelmed or to run aimlessly to find some sort of answer. Instead, more than ever, you need to stop what you are doing, take a deep breath, and seek the Father. Scripture makes it clear that when you approach God with an open and pure heart, asking for wisdom, He provides it. God wants to help provide peace and clarity as you make decisions. This doesn't mean that the fatigue will no longer be present, but that you will have a clear mind to make the decision that you need to make.

Don't put the pressure on yourself to know what to do in your own ability. Don't rely on your own power and strength to make the decision. Rely on the wisdom that God provides and the strength that God supplies!

QUESTIONS TO CONSIDER:

- What is your natural response when you become drained from making decisions? (Anger, feel hopeless, lash out at those around you, run away from responsibility)

- At the core of it, why do you think you respond in that way?

- Next time you find yourself in this situation, what can you do to help you remember James 1:5?

TAKEAWAY:

Say this prayer: God, I am worn down from life and making decisions. In my own power, I cannot keep this up. Please give me wisdom on the decisions I need to make in my life. Help me have clarity and peace during the entire process. Thank You for always providing what I need. Amen.

DAY 21: EAST TO WEST

GOD'S WORD:

If we confess our sins, he is faithful and just and will forgive us our sins and purify us from all unrighteousness.

1 John 1:9

TODAY'S THOUGHT:

Let me throw a made-up scenario your way. What if I was physically chained to a pillar for years? I couldn't go anywhere. I couldn't do anything. I was forced to stay in one spot, chained. (I know, weird scenario, but hear me out.) Every day, I would see the chains and would be reminded of how they were holding me back. Of course, that would be torture. But what if finally, one day someone comes to my rescue with keys in hand, unlocking the chains, which no longer bind me to that post. The appropriate response would be to say *"thank you"* and joyfully skip away. But what if I just stayed there? What if I questioned if I was really set free, saying, *"It looks like the chains are unlocked, but maybe it did not really happen. I guess I'll just stay here in this same spot as I have been for the past years."* That would be crazy. Hopefully, no one would choose to do that.

The sad reality is that we often do that regarding our sin. Bondage is the result of sin. Our mistakes, failures, sins leave us chained and full of regret. The way to find freedom is no secret. It is through accepting the gift of salvation from God. In that moment, your sins are forgiven, Christ comes into your life, and unlocks the chains of bondage. For some reason, though, there is a tendency to still allow those chains and mistakes to rule over us. We still hold onto past regret, believing that real freedom is too good to be true. Remaining a slave to our sin leads to diminished mental health, never fully moving on to grow, never living a life of joy or bringing glory to God. I do not want that for your life.

God is not holding a piece of paper with your name on it, writing every sin you commit in permanent marker. I like to think that He is writing in pencil and once you seek forgiveness and He forgives you, He takes out a big eraser and wipes the record of that sin away. He doesn't hold it over your head or just mark a line through it to where you can still see it. He wipes it clean. Psalms 103:12 says, *"As far as the east is from the west, so far has he removed our transgressions from us."* When traveling east or west, there is no starting or ending point. It's simply never ending. If you have asked for forgiveness, God has forgiven you. He has taken that eraser and removed it. Stop holding onto something that God is not. Your mistakes do not have to rule over your life. Your chains do not have to stay on. Those chains only have power over you if you allow them to.

QUESTIONS TO CONSIDER:

- Do you struggle to believe that God really has forgiven all of your sins? Do you tend to look back at your past sin as if it defines you in some way?

- How would your thinking change if you truly believed God cast your sins as far as the east is from the west? In what ways would your mental health be improved in doing so?

TAKEAWAY:

Say this prayer: God, help me to believe the truth that You do not hold my past sins against me. I will no longer stay chained in bondage, since those chains do not have power over me. I will be free in You today! Amen.

DAY 22: BOTTLE OF TEARS

You have kept count of my tossings; put my tears in your bottle.
Are they not in your book?

Psalms 56:8 (ESV)

TODAY'S THOUGHT:

Some days you cannot help but cry. The weight of mental illness is a heavy load to bear. It can feel overwhelming every day to be where you need to be, do what you need to do, extend your relational energy, and be present, all while your mental illness is hanging above your head like a cloud. By the time you make it to the end of the day, you are drained mentally, physically, and emotionally. The result is tears running down your cheeks, sometimes uncontrollably.

Do not worry, you are in good company. David, one of the most respected men in the Bible, was very open about the tears he shed. In the biblical account for today, David was forced to flee to an enemy city to escape death. He found himself in a difficult, isolating time. As he often did, David continuously prayed to God and reflected on the numerous occasions where he had fallen face down and cried out to Him. David had always shared every emotion with God, and was confident that God knew every tear he had shed. Tears in a bottle (which is not a remix to *Message in a Bottle*) may sound strange to you, but David had a reason for saying it. Archaeologists have discovered small "tear bottles" that were used by those mourning to collect their tears, so that they could lay the bottle at the grave.[8] David was implying that God was watching his life so intently, that He preserved David's tears and placed them in a bottle.

With that being said, let the tears roll. It is okay to cry. It is okay to be honest in the moment and acknowledge you feel stretched thin. Crying out to God does not make you weak. It makes you human. Like David, you can know with confidence that your tears do not go unnoticed. God knows when you cry. He understands your suffering and the toll your mental health is taking. He is, in a sense, collecting your bottle of tears. You are not alone. But know that the time of crying will come to an end. Ecclesiastes 3:4 says there is *a time to weep and a time to laugh.*" You will not always feel the way you feel right now. You will experience laughter and enjoyment, as God fills you with His joy.

QUESTIONS TO CONSIDER:

- Do you feel alone when you cry; that your tears go unnoticed? Why or why not?

- What does it bring to your life, knowing that God is aware of your tears? (security, comfort, peace, etc.)

- What can you do or put into place to make sure you remember these truths when you find yourself in a time of crying out?

TAKEAWAY:

Say this prayer: God, at times, I feel so alone when I am overwhelmed. I want to know with confidence that You see my tears and understand how I feel. I ask for your comfort during those times. You have made it clear that they will not last forever. Amen.

---

[8] Warren Wiersbe, *The Wiersbe Bible Commentary*, OT (Colorado Springs: David C. Cook, 2007), 939.

DAY 23: VICTORY IN THE MIDST OF PAIN

GOD'S WORD:

The LORD gives strength to his people;
the LORD blesses his people with peace.
Psalms 29:11

TODAY'S THOUGHT:

Your fight against mental illness can feel like a never-ending battle. It can feel like more defeat than victory. More anxiety than rest. More stress than relaxation. More worry than peace. More low days than high days. Mental illness can leave you wondering if you have what it takes to keep going on. Can you ever find victory in it?

As I write this, I am in the midst of pain and uncertainty. Many days feel like I am losing. I have wrestled with the question of when and if I will find victory over this battle of mental illness. What I discovered is that I was looking through the wrong perspective. I was not being realistic in the way I defined it. I found that we have to redefine what victory looks like and when it is accomplished. Victory can, but does not have to, look like mental illness magically disappearing out of your life completely. Instead, victory is living your life in a way that you are healthy and joyful, while having mental illness. It is found in managing your health and not allowing mental illness to call the shots. Victory is not a one-time occurrence. It does not only come at the end of your life. It's an ongoing process. There is victory to be found every day in Christ.

49

I am seeing that, even in the midst of this difficult journey, I am finding victories. Mental illness does not have to completely disappear out of my life for me to hold my hands up as the victor. Every day, I now want to build on top of my prior wins. God wants to not only give His people peace, but He wants to give strength. It is through His strength that you are able to manage your mental illness to find victory. Victory *can* be found in the midst of your pain, hardships, and struggles.

Questions To Consider:

- Look back at the past few days: were you able to manage your mental health any of those days? If so, then you have victories to build upon!

- How will this perspective help you today?

- What are ways that you have been able to manage your mental health?

Takeaway:

Say this prayer: Lord, I know I do not have to experience defeat in my mental health. I need Your peace and strength in my life. I know You want to supply those to me as I look to You. Help me find victory in the midst of my pain. Amen.

DAY 24: VIEW OF GOD

GOD'S WORD:

Ask and it will be given to you; seek and you will find; knock and the door will be opened to you. For everyone who asks receives; the one who seeks finds; and to the one who knocks, the door will be opened.

Matthew 7:7–8

TODAY'S THOUGHT:

One of the most powerful quotes I have ever heard comes from A.W. Tozer, *"What comes to your mind when you think about God is the most important thing about you."*[9]

Chip Ingram, a pastor and author, explains it in a unique way. He asked the question, "What's Your First Domino?"[10] Each one of us has a first domino. It is what makes us who we are. It affects the other aspects of our life. It affects the foundation of your marriage, the conversations you have, the decisions you make, the way you view situations around you, the way you view your mental illness. Everything is based off of the first domino. Your first domino, whether you realize it or not, is your *view of God.* Deep down in your core, you naturally gravitate toward your mental image of God. Everything is rooted in that perception of God. That can be a scary or comforting reality.

There is good news. You can bring clarity to your view of God as you grow in Him. The more you get into the Word of God, learn about

---

[9] "A.W. Tozer Quotes," Good Reads, accessed November 1, 2020, https://www.goodreads.com/author/quotes/1082290.A_W_Tozer.

[10] Chip Ingram, "What's Your First Domino?" *Rightnow Conference*, Orlando, Florida, 2018, https://www. rightnowmedia.org/Content/Series/294128?episode=6.

Him, His attributes, His truths, the clearer the picture of God becomes. That is His desire. He wants a deeper, more intimate relationship with you. Scripture promises if you seek God wanting to see Him accurately, He will make Himself known to you. He will give you a fuller picture of who He is.

QUESTIONS TO CONSIDER:

- How do you currently view God? Do you think you tend to focus on one of God's attributes more than the others? For example: His love, faithfulness, goodness, justice, wisdom.

- Can you see that if you only focused on that one attribute how it wouldn't give a full, accurate picture of who God is and how He works?

TAKEAWAY:

Say this prayer: Lord, help me see You clearer. I want to have an accurate picture of You. I yearn to get into Your Word to learn and understand Your attributes. Amen.

DAY 25: GOD'S LOVE NOTE

GOD'S WORD:

For the word of God is alive and active. Sharper than any double-edged sword, it penetrates even to dividing soul and spirit, joints and marrow; it judges the thoughts and attitudes of the heart.

Hebrews 4:12

TODAY'S THOUGHT:

Charles H. Spurgeon said, *"If you wish to know God, you must know His Word. If you wish to perceive His power, you must see how He works by His Word. If you wish to know His purpose before it comes to pass, you can only discover it by His Word."* [11].

It was the summer of 2012. My wife, Jessica, and I had just started dating and were in the young puppy love stage. And before I get in trouble, we still are! During that summer, we had been able to see each other several times each week. But that was going to change, as I was heading out to lead worship for a camp. Jessica wrote me a letter for each day while I was at camp. When she handed me the letters, my game plan was to read all of them on the first day, but she had guidelines for me. I was only to read the letter assigned for that day. That seemed easy enough, until I read that first love note and then all I wanted to do was to read the rest. The mystery of what she wrote for each of the other days was consuming me. But I knew I made Jessica a promise. Each morning, as soon as my alarm went off, the first thing I did was read Jessica's love note. I was fascinated with

---

[11] "Charles Spurgeon Quotes about Purpose," AZ Quotes, accessed November 1, 2020, https://www.azquotes.com/author/13978-Charles_Spurgeon/tag/purpose

learning new things about her. Her words weren't boring or stale; there was life in each word. There was something about the way she would end each letter with "*I love you*" that brought a smile to my face.

It was Jessica's love notes that helped me realize that the way I approached the Bible was shallow and insignificant. The Bible isn't just any book, it is THE book. These are the Words of God. When God speaks, big things happen. He spoke and the universe was created, everything we see around us and beyond.

The Word of God is *active*. It is full of *life*. It *speaks* to your innermost being. If you will read with an eager and open heart, God will reveal Himself and His character to you. He will bring to your attention things in your life that you may not have realized. What better way to get to know God and who He is, than by reading His Words? Through His Word, God tells you that He loves you and that He is all you will ever need. Wow. Talk about a *real* love note.

QUESTIONS TO CONSIDER:

- How have you viewed the Bible in the past? Do you read it expecting God to speak to you?

- What can you do to make sure you spend time in the Word of God each week?

TAKEAWAY:

Pre-determine the place, time, and which part of the Bible you will read. An option for your quiet time could be to expand on the verse of the day from this devotional. You could read the verses around it or the entire chapter.

DAY 26: SHINE A LIGHT

GOD'S WORD:

Your word is a lamp for my feet, a light on my path.

Psalms 119:105

TODAY'S THOUGHT:

King David refers to God's Word as a light. When David was writing this, he didn't have a floodlight. He didn't have a light switch that he could flip on. He definitely didn't have the cool set-up to clap and the lights turn on for the room. He had a lamp, which didn't light up everything in the room. It provided just enough light for a few steps ahead of him.[12] He was dependent on that light to walk through the room, eat food, do what he needed to do. It is that picture that he uses to compare to God's Word. As he read God's Words, it would shine a light for the next step he was to take. As he took a couple of steps in that direction and continued to hear God's truths, the next couple of steps would light up.

As you manage your mental health, there will never be a time in your life that you won't need a light to help provide direction. You will always need guidance. God's Word is not a light that reveals all things, but it does reveal enough light for us to walk through a dark world, in the ways of God.

Look to the Bible to shine a light, guiding you where to step next. Let it provide direction. If you read the Bible, but don't act on what you read, you are just standing still in the dark. What good is it to

---

[12] The reThink Group, Inc., "The Word of God is a Light that Directs Our Path," *XP3 On the Lot (1) Lights!* (January 2008): 8.

shine a light if you don't step in the direction of the light? Read God's Word, let it shine, and then step where it shines.

QUESTIONS TO CONSIDER:

- Will you allow God's Word to be a lamp that lights up your path as you walk through this dark world?

- Will you take the Word of God seriously enough to spend time with it throughout the week?

- What is one step you can take today to make sure you spend time in God's Word?

TAKEAWAY:

Say this prayer: God, I need Your Word to direct my steps. If I try to lead on my own, I always end up tripping in the dark. Please open my eyes to where You are shining. Thank You for Your Word. Amen.

DAY 27: HIDE AND SEEK

GOD'S WORD:

I have hidden your word in my heart that I might not sin against you.

Psalms 119:11

TODAY'S THOUGHT:

When I was in seminary, I took a class with a professor named Dr. Max Barnett. God really spoke to me through Dr. Barnett. He was a man who had been following the Lord for a long time and it was evident in the way he spoke, listened, and acted. He shared with the class how Scripture memory had changed his life. He said that memorizing God's Word is taking seriously what God says. When God's Word is in your heart, you can bring it to the forefront of your mind at any moment.

Scripture memory is extremely valuable whether you have an opportunity to share about God's love with someone, if you're tempted with something you know you shouldn't do, or if you need encouragement to keep moving forward with your mental illness. Those days that you feel defeat, extreme anxiety, or collapsing depression, you need the Word of God available to be spoken into your life.

Here's the thing...memorizing Scripture can seem intimidating, but memorizing one verse every two weeks is very doable. Throughout the week, you have a lot of extra minutes. A couple of minutes walking to your car. Fifteen minutes waiting in the doctor's office. Several minutes waiting for your coffee at the coffee shop. If you review the Bible verse that you are memorizing for even a couple of minutes every day for two weeks, you should have no problem memorizing that verse. If you did that every two weeks, by the end of the year, you would have 26 verses memorized. 26 verses, the sacred Words of God, stored away in your heart and mind, reminding you of the truths of God. That is powerful.

QUESTIONS TO CONSIDER:

- In your life, what is the scenario that comes up where you desperately need Scripture to come to mind the most?

- Will you look up which verses speak truth in those situations and start with those?

TAKEAWAY:

I believe one of the best methods for consistent Scripture memorizing is a memory verse holder, a pack which holds the verse that you are currently memorizing. It also holds past verses you have learned, so that you can keep refreshing your memory on those, as well. You can order a memory verse pack online or simply use index cards with a rubber band. I challenge you to begin by memorizing Romans 15:13, a powerful verse about hope.

DAY 28: HEARING THE WHISPER

GOD'S WORD:

Coming over to us, he took Paul's belt, tied his own hands and feet with it
and said, "The Holy Spirit says, 'In this way the Jewish leaders in
Jerusalem will bind the owner of this belt and will hand him over to the
Gentiles.' " When we heard this, we and the people there pleaded with Paul
not to go up to Jerusalem. Then Paul answered, "Why are you weeping and
breaking my heart? I am ready not only to be bound, but also to die in
Jerusalem for the name of the Lord Jesus."

Acts 21:11–13

TODAY'S THOUGHT:

If you are like me on most days, you would sum up life in one
word...busy. Life can be chaotic and loud. Busyness creates noise.
There is always something to do, somewhere to be, someone to tend
to. The addition of mental illness only magnifies the chaos. You might
say that you are maxed out on the amount of volume you can handle
in your life. During these busy times, you and I need to be able to
hear the voice of God for guidance and direction. What I have seen to
be true, though, is that rarely does God speak with a booming audible
voice or through a burning bush or by a writing hand on the wall.
God often chooses to speak through a quiet whisper; the opposite of
the chaotic noise that is all around.

In today's verses, a prophet, named Agabus, stopped Paul on his
missionary journey to warn him that if he continued on to Jerusalem
to preach the gospel, he would be taken, bound, and persecuted.
Paul's friends urged him to turn around and not risk his life. This did
not faze Paul, though. Even after all of this, Paul held to his belief

that God had instructed him to continue on, despite the upcoming persecution. The world was screaming in Paul's ear to stay, but on the other hand, God was quietly whispering, "Go." How did Paul hear the whisper in the chaos and noise? Let me answer that question with a story.

I played high school basketball and would often practice in the afternoons with my dad. We would spend quite a bit of time on the worst part of my game...free throws. Shaquille O'Neal and I probably had the same free throw percentage. My dad would help me with my form, my follow through, positioning my feet. One game during the season, all of my practice was tested. I was fouled in the last couple of minutes of a close game, meaning I would have to face my worst enemy: the free throw line. The gymnasium was filled with people screaming. It was loud. It was chaotic. It would have been easy to listen to everyone yelling. Instead of doing that, though, I decided to look to the man that I had spent night after night practicing free throws with. As I looked to my dad, I saw him make the motion with his hands that we had practiced over and over and his lips mouthing the words, "Follow through." Because I had spent so much time with my dad, it was easy to listen to his whisper over the yells of the crowd.

I believe in the same way, Paul had spent so much time in the presence of God, seeking His voice, it was not difficult to hear God's whisper in the midst of the world yelling. You see, *until you spend time with God in the quiet, you can't expect to hear Him in the chaos.* Without you getting away to focus solely on God, spending time in His Word, communicating with Him, you may never hear Him whisper. The last thing I want is for you is to miss out on what God desires to do IN you, THROUGH you, and AROUND you. Now I know you may be wondering if I made the free throws, but that isn't important. That is not the aspect of the story we need to focus on. Okay, I didn't make the free throws. Let's move on to the next section!

Questions To Consider:

- Are you in a busy season right now? If so, does it feel impossible to hear God?

- When life gets chaotic, do you tend to run to God or try to handle everything yourself?

- What changes do you need to make to spend time with God?

Takeaway:

Say this prayer: Lord, I want to hear Your voice every day. I want to spend so much time with You on a regular basis that I look to You at all times. Help me listen for Your voice, instead of the world. I love You. Amen.

Until you spend time with God in the quiet,
you can't expect to hear Him in the chaos.

DAY 29: A HEALTHY, HAPPY YOU

GOD'S WORD:

The thief comes only to steal and kill and destroy; I have come that they may have life, and have it to the full.

John 10:10

TODAY'S THOUGHT:

I want to start with a statement that you may not hear or think about very often...*God wants you to be joy filled.* That is such a simple statement, but it seems almost too good to be true. But if God really does want us to be filled with joy, then why is it so hard to be joyful? Well, I think we are confusing living in a fallen world with what God wants for us. God wants you to enjoy life; to enjoy it to the fullest, actually. He made you to enjoy His creation. That is why He gave you passions, interests, hobbies. This verse indicates that believers actually have the opportunity to be the most joyful people on earth...that doesn't exclude those battling mental illness! The reason is because true joy comes from an overflow of Jesus in your life.

That goes hand-in-hand with the fact that God wants you to be healthy. You have a part in that. There is already evidence that you are taking this topic seriously, since you are going through this book. One of the goals of this book is to learn how to best manage your mental health (huge praise if the mental illness is ever taken away completely.) You deserve to enjoy life. You deserve to be healthy. The mental illness is there, but it doesn't have to steal your joy.

Do you know what this means? You can do your hobbies without feeling guilty. You need to pursue your passions. You ought to celebrate life with a fun activity as often as possible. Why else would God give you those interests and passions? I 100% believe that you can live a joyful life in the midst of mental illness. It will take intentionality daily, focusing your eyes on Christ, and making wise decisions, but it will be worth it tenfold!

QUESTIONS TO CONSIDER:

- Do you struggle to find joy? If so, what is the obstacle?
- Do you believe that God really does want you to be joy filled?
- What might this change of perspective do for your life?

TAKEAWAY:

Say this prayer: Lord, change my perspective today. I know You want me to enjoy life and enjoy it to the fullest. Please allow Your joy and love to overflow out of my life. Amen.

DAY 30: WHAT'S FEAR GOT TO DO WITH IT?

GOD'S WORD:

So do not fear, for I am with you;
do not be dismayed, for I am your God.
I will strengthen you and help you;
I will uphold you with my righteous right hand.

Isaiah 41:1

TODAY'S THOUGHT:

Moana, the Disney movie released in 2016, has been watched in my household numerous times. In the movie, Moana overcomes fear to sail across the open sea on a mission to save her people and her island. At one point in the movie, she says, *"Sometimes our strengths lie beneath the surface. Far beneath, in some cases."*[13] I agree with her statement, but not necessarily in the way she intended it. Moana was referring to inner strength that comes from yourself. You and I do find strength beneath the surface, but that strength doesn't come from us; it comes from the Lord.

Fear is a powerful emotion. When used to the right degree, with the right purpose, it is beneficial to warn against potential harm. But when taken to an extreme or when it begins to constantly linger, it becomes crippling and can even become life-altering. Fear can become one of the biggest robbers of joy. The more you believe the

---

[13]Ron Clements, John Musker, Chris Williams, and Don Hall. *Moana*. (2016; United States: Walt Disney Studios Motion Pictures.)

lies of fear, the more it taints your perspective of life, especially if you are taking on new responsibilities, walking into unknown territory and situations, or battling hardships. No one wants to live their lives with an unhealthy fear. But if you were to really examine your life, you may say that you view your mental illness in a fearful way. At times, it can feel like it's too overwhelming. But the truth is that fear does not have to overcome you.

God knew how big of a deal fear would be, so the phrase *"Fear Not"* appears in the Bible 365 times...once for every day of the year! When something is repeated, it usually means it is pretty important. God definitely wanted you to know that you do not have to be afraid. Whether you realize it or not, during every circumstance and difficulty that you will endure, God is right there with you. You are not walking through it alone. Not only is God with you, but He has promised to not allow it to overcome you. His presence is what equips you to have courage and overcome fear in your life.

Pastor and author, Crawford Loritts said, *"Courage doesn't mean that I am not afraid. It means that I fear God more than I fear my environment. It means that I trust in divine resources more than the resources of man."*[14] As you look out on the open sea of the adventure of today, have confidence that God will equip you and strengthen you with HIS power!

Questions To Consider:

- What are you most fearful of right now? Where does that fear come from?

- What can you do this week to remind you to *fear not*?

---

[14]Crawford Loritts, "The Call to Courage," accessed October 10, 2020, https://preachingchristos.wordpress.com/2017/03/10/the-call-to-courage-by-craw ford-loritts-joshua-11-9/.

TAKEAWAY:

At some point today, listen to the song *"Our God"*[15] by Chris Tomlin. The bridge of the song highlights the powerful verse, Romans 8:31, *"What, then, shall we say in response to these things? If God is for us, who can be against us?"* Let's make this our anthem today.

---

[15] Chris Tomlin, "Our God," *And If Our God is For Us*, Sparrow Records, 2010. *Youtube, youtu.be/NJpt1hSYf2o.*

The phrase "Fear Not" appears in the Bible 365 times...
once for every day of the year!

DAY 31: WRONG QUESTIONS, WRONG ANSWERS?

GOD'S WORD:

As he went along, he saw a man blind from birth. His disciples asked him,
"Rabbi, who sinned, this man or his parents, that he was born blind?"
"Neither this man nor his parents sinned," said Jesus, "but this happened so
that the works of God might be displayed in him."

John 9:1–3

TODAY'S THOUGHT:

I remember several occasions when my math teacher would tell me
something close to *"You are asking the wrong question. You need to
look at the problem from a different perspective to get the right answer."*
Because I was stubborn, I was stuck looking at the equation in the
wrong way. It was leading me nowhere. John Capozzi explains it,
"To get the right answer, it helps to ask the right question."[16] It doesn't
matter the number of times you ask the question; if it's the wrong
question, you will always fall short of finding the right answer. This
only leads to frustration and uncertainty.

Too often, we continually ask God the wrong question and wonder
why He is not answering us or providing the solution we desire. For
me, I can get stuck on the questions of *"Why do I have to suffer with
depression and anxiety, God? Why will you not take it away from me
completely?"* You may have cried out to God with similar questions

---

[16] "Right Answer Quotes," AZ Quotes, accessed October 3, 2021,
https://www.azquotes.com/quotes/topics/right-answers.html.

about your pain. You ask once, twice, three times; maybe even tweak the way you ask it, but it feels as if God will not reveal the answer or He does not hear you. While God wants us to communicate with Him how we feel at all times, we could be asking the wrong question. We might be looking at the problem from the wrong perspective.

What if God is wanting to draw others to Himself through your pain? What if God has already planned out an extraordinary display of His love to the world through your struggles and difficult circumstances? The Bible is full of examples of God doing just that. In today's passage, the disciples were looking from the wrong perspective and, as a result, asked the wrong question. The man was not blind because of anyone's sin, but so that God's glory could be shown. Do not allow your painful experience or your mental illness to taint your view of God or what He is trying to do in and through your life. Begin asking God how He is wanting to draw others to Himself through your pain. Why? Because, if you want *"to get the right answer, it helps to ask the right question."*

QUESTIONS TO CONSIDER:

- Do you get stuck on wondering why you are having to suffer or experience certain pain? Why or why not?

- Look at your current pain: what specific things might God want to do through it?

TAKEAWAY:

Say this prayer: God, I want to start asking the right questions. I do not want to view my life in regard to only myself. Please use my life, pain, and experiences for Your glory. Draw people to You through me. Amen.

DAY 32: THANKFULNESS

God's Word:

*Let the peace of Christ rule in your hearts, since as members of one body
you were called to peace. And be thankful.*

Colossians 3:15

Today's Thought:

There is a real sense of entitlement in the United States of America (I'm
sure that applies to other countries, as well). You may find yourself
in the routine of focusing on the one or two things that you're not
totally happy with and by doing so, neglect the numerous things that
you do have to be thankful for. If you and I aren't careful with this, it
can lead to us becoming numb, bitter, greedy, discontent, and envying
others. When you spend your time being ungrateful, whether it is
intentional or not, it can become a barrier to God working in your life.
You begin to miss out on the times that God wants to reveal Himself
to you or teach you something new, because your focus is elsewhere.

Being grateful frees you from comparisons and unrealistic expectations. It is the cure to discontentment. It's impossible to truly
be grateful and discontent in the same moment. This is a process;
contentment does not come right away. It's a discipline you learn,
not a feeling you experience. The more you give thanks to God, the
more you will see all of the things you have to be thankful for.

When I begin to focus on my battles with anxiety and depression,
wondering why I have to deal with them, I now know to stop what
I'm doing and refocus my attention. In these moments, you and I
have to choose contentment; to focus on everything we have to be
thankful for (which I'm sure is more than we can even count!)

QUESTIONS TO CONSIDER:

Read Psalms 100:1–5 and then reflect on the following questions:

- Is being thankful a struggle for you?
- Do you truly believe that you have plenty to be grateful for?
- Will you choose the discipline of contentment?

TAKEAWAY:

Grab a piece of paper and pen and make a *thankful list*. Write out every single person, gift, talent, passion, possession, food, clothing item, and so on, that you have to be thankful for. I am always surprised at how long my list is each time I do this activity. You can pull out this list on days when you struggle to be thankful.

DAY 33: DON'T STAY IN ISOLATION

GOD'S WORD:

*Consequently, you are no longer foreigners and strangers, but fellow
citizens with God's people and also members of his household, built on the
foundation of the apostles and prophets, with Christ Jesus himself as the
chief cornerstone. In him the whole building is joined together and rises to
become a holy temple in the Lord. And in him you too are being built
together to become a dwelling in which God lives by his Spirit.*
Ephesians 2:19–22

TODAY'S THOUGHT:

Have you ever heard of the redwood tree? They are commonly found
along the coast of northern California. Redwood trees are massive
trees, standing hundreds of feet tall. Anyone would assume that a
350-foot-tall tree would require deep roots, but that's not the case for
this tree. The redwood tree roots are actually very shallow, usually 5
or 6 feet deep. But they make up for it in width, sometimes extending
out 100 feet from the trunk. They thrive in thick groves, where the
roots from all the Redwood trees fuse together and intertwine. By
doing so, they can withstand high winds and raging floods, because
of the strength the trees have together. Each tree is stronger because
it is surrounded and intertwined by a grove, a community of other
redwood trees. That is not by accident. God designed the redwood
trees to function in that way.

Naturally, when you face dark periods, or frequent lows and highs,
the tendency is to pull away from everything and everyone. Being
around other people and having to explain what is going on seems
like more work, with little benefit. But long periods of isolation are

a very dangerous thing. In those moments you're in a weaker state, fighting against your mind, which doesn't always tell the truth. Your mind can start to convince you of lies and of worst-case scenarios. The longer that it goes on, the more alone you feel. It's especially important in the dark times and low periods, to have a community, a grove, people to lock arms with. Having people who have your best interest in mind are not just for the happier times, they are there to help you in the valley. They are there to get into the boxing ring with you. Oftentimes, we just keep them at arm's length and then wonder why we feel isolated. God designed the Christian life to always be lived with other believers. He knew that we would need each other and that we would function best when intertwined with a community of believers.

The word *"church"* comes from the Greek word *"ekklesia"* which is a general term referring to a gathering or assembly. So, when you read the word *"ekklesia"* (church) in the Bible, you know it's referring to a gathering. It's a family to grow with. God built His church with Jesus as the cornerstone and believers as the body of Christ. You need others to pick you up when you fall to remind you of God's truth and to enjoy life with you. There is something different about going through life with the people of Jesus. In those rough periods, don't pull away. Don't try to live in isolation. Instead, lean into Christ and the people that He has placed around you. Because, in Christ, *you too are being built together to become a dwelling in which God lives by His Spirit.*

QUESTIONS TO CONSIDER:

- Do you tend to pull away from others when your mental illness gets worse? How can you prevent that from happening?

- Are you involved in a church? Do you have a community of believers? If not, I urge you to find a group and be a part of it.

Takeaway:

Say this prayer: Lord, thank You for designing the church in a way that relationships are vitally important. I know the church is there to help me grow in all areas of life. Help me lean into the resources You have given me when times get tough. Amen.

It's especially important in the dark times and low periods,
to have a community, a grove, people to lock arms with.

DAY 34: SNOWFLAKES AND FINGERPRINTS

GOD'S WORD:

For you created my inmost being; you knit me together in my mother's womb. I praise you because I am fearfully and wonderfully made; your works are wonderful, I know that full well.

Psalms 139:13–14

TODAY'S THOUGHT:

I'm sure you have heard that no two snowflakes are the same and that no two human fingerprints are identical either. While this may come as common knowledge to you, it is rather significant and worth pointing out for today's thought.

You are bound to have days when the world seems so dark and hopeless that you don't feel you have enough strength to carry on. The thought might enter your mind that it would be better if life on earth came to a stop for you. First of all, if that is where you find yourself right now, my heart aches for you. My inner being longs to encourage you in any way possible. I know how heavy that burden can be, and it's a miserable state to be in. I ask you out of the sincerest love to read this next part and really aim to believe it deep down.

No matter how difficult it gets in your mind, please hold on. This world needs you. There is so much more beauty ahead of you, that maybe you just can't see yet. Your life is incredibly valuable. God knew everything about you long before He ever created you. He delicately wired you and made you exactly how He wanted to. You're loved in a deeper sense than the human mind can comprehend. God loved you enough that He went the most extreme measure, sending His Son to the cross, just so you could have a relationship with Him and find forgiveness for your sins.

When you are tired of fighting, hold on; you are immensely *valuable.*

When you feel hopeless, hold on; you are *irreplaceable.*

When you wonder the purpose of continuing, hold on; you are deeply *loved.*

There is no one else like you and that is a wonderful thing. God made the perfect *you.* The world needs your snowflake. Those around you need your fingerprint. You have to keep your mind focused on the day ahead of you, and then the next, and the next. Allow the strength of God and the resources around you to keep moving you forward.

Questions To Consider:

- Is this a regular battle for you? Do you dwell on these kinds of thoughts consistently?

- Do you have people you can reach out to when needed? Who is that?

- Have you tried other resources as well: doctor visit, counseling, so on? If not, would you consider checking out those resources?

Takeaway:

If you answered *'yes'* to the first question, text or call a trusted person today and tell them about today's devotional and ask for any type of help that you need. At any point, you can reach out to the National Suicide Prevention Lifeline at 800-273-8255.

DAY 35: COMMUNICATION, COMMUNICATION, COMMUNICATION

GOD'S WORD:

Two are better than one, because they have a good return for their labor: If either of them falls down, one can help the other up. But pity anyone who falls and has no one to help them up.

Ecclesiastes 4:9–10

TODAY'S THOUGHT:

You may assume that the people around you don't truly care about you or want what is best for you, because they aren't responding to your mental illness in the way you need. I have felt like that many times, as well. We have to take a step back and realize that even someone who deals with mental illness has trouble understanding what someone with a different aspect of mental illness is battling. If that's the case, then someone who doesn't deal with mental illness at all is going to have an extremely difficult time understanding. It's a whole different world and doesn't usually make sense to them.

I have good news, though. If that's how you feel, there is hope. If you are the one on the other side, who doesn't battle ongoing mental illness, there is hope to better the situation. It comes down to communication, communication, communication. There has to be a willingness to have very open and real discussions, even if it's painful to bring up some of those dark times.

The more your loved one is able to understand what you feel, what you are thinking, how life's circumstances are affecting you, the more they can support you. The more they begin to understand what it looks like to walk in your shoes, the more they can display their love for you. Clarity and understanding enter the picture. The transition to proper aid and support begins. It starts, though, with you choosing to be open and choosing to share as much as you can, even if it's difficult to talk about. Remember, they may simply not understand what you are walking through. Don't allow a lack of communication to become a barrier.

Questions To Consider:

- Do you tend to bottle up what you feel because you believe people don't care or won't understand? If so, what has that been doing to you?

- Are you willing to open up to a loved one? Who do you need to talk to first?

Takeaway:

Say this prayer: God, I know I can't walk this journey alone. I need You and I need the people around me. Help me put down my pride, guilt, or anything holding me back from trusting You and other believers around me. Amen.

DAY 36: SUNRISE TO SUNSET

GOD'S WORD:

Praise the LORD. Praise the LORD, you his servants; praise the name of the LORD. Let the name of the LORD be praised, both now and forevermore. From the rising of the sun to the place where it sets, the name of the LORD is to be praised.

Psalms 113:1–3

TODAY'S THOUGHT:

There is not a limit to the number of times a sunrise or sunset will take your breath away. It is always a beautiful sight to see. I have never watched the sunset and thought, *"That is bland, boring, and ugly."* Something else that I have found to be true is that the sun seems to set and rise on a steady basis. Every morning and night, the sun stays on schedule, letting you know that the day is starting, or the day is ending. The number of days, all around the world, that the sun rises and sets is the amount of days that God is to be praised. I will help you out in case you drifted off...that means every single day. Warren Wiersbe said, *"This kind of praise pays no attention to time ("forever more") or space (from east to west)."*[17] There should not be a day that goes by where you do not give praise to the Creator of the universe.

If you are not careful, you can find yourself praising God only when everything falls into place. But this verse does not say only praise God some days. Instead, no matter how smooth or rough the

---

[17]Warren Wiersbe, *The Wiersbe Bible Commentary*, NT (Colorado Springs: David C. Cook, 2007), 999.

day is going; God should be worshipped. When the kids are listening or when they drive you crazy. When you excel in your job or when you get passed over for the promotion. When you pass your big exam or when you fail part of it. When you get a good report from the doctor or when the results do not come back how you hoped. When your mental health is in a healthy place or when it takes a dive down. In ALL circumstances, at ALL times, God is always good and worthy of your admiration, praise, honor. How you feel about life's circumstances will change consistently, but God will never change.

From now on, when you see a sunrise or sunset, let it remind you to praise the One who made it all.

QUESTIONS TO CONSIDER:

- If you examine your life, when do you find yourself praising God the most? The least? Why is that?

- How would praising God in the low moments of life change your perspective and heart?

TAKEAWAY:

In these specific verses, the word "name" is used three times to refer to God's character, who He is, and what He does. Pick two attributes of God and spend a moment praising Him for those attributes. (Some of God's attributes are His faithfulness, wisdom, mercy, justice, love.)

DAY 37: A TIME OF HEALING

GOD'S WORD:

*Some men came carrying a paralyzed man on a mat and tried to take him
into the house to lay him before Jesus. When they could not find a way to
do this because of the crowd, they went up on the roof and lowered him on
his mat through the tiles into the middle of the crowd, right in front of
Jesus...So he said to the paralyzed man, "I tell you, get up, take your mat
and go home." Immediately he stood up in front of them, took what he had
been lying on and went home praising God.*

Luke 5:18–25

TODAY'S THOUGHT:

After getting to a place where I felt like I couldn't continue on and
then stepping away from my job, I knew if there was anything that I
needed, it was *healing*. I felt like I had been beaten up by life. I felt
like it had taken a toll on my mental and emotional health, leaving
me broken. I didn't need a new adventure to jump into or a new
job to simply get my mind off of things. I needed healing. I needed
restoration. As I write this, I'm still in that place and I'm committed
to seek healing for as long as it takes.

You might be there, too. You might be in a broken state, in need
of healing. What God has been revealing to me in this season is that
true healing for my soul can only come from one place...Him. There
are a lot of other things in this world that can temporarily take away
pain or capture my attention, but they quickly fade away. There's
only one source of healing and it's the arms of Christ.

The first step is to realize your need for Jesus. You have to tear
down any walls that were built up over the years of pretending that

everything was okay. Instead of turning to the earthly things at arm's reach, you have to humble yourself and admit you need help from the only One who can truly bring healing, Jesus.

The next step is to simply go; go to Christ. Spend time in the quietness with God. Read His Word. Pray as often as you can. Listen to worship music. You will be surprised at how much God has to share with you and how He desires to heal your soul. It is only when you turn to Jesus that you find true healing.

QUESTIONS TO CONSIDER:

- Are you in need of healing? What kind of healing?
- What is holding you back from going to the arms of Christ?

TAKEAWAY:

Say this prayer: Lord, I desperately need healing. I need restoration. I will run to Your arms and find everything I need there. Thank You for accepting me just as I am. I love You. Amen.

DAY 38: I KNOW I NEED TO SAY NO

GOD'S WORD:

At daybreak, Jesus went out to a solitary place. The people were looking for him and when they came to where he was, they tried to keep him from leaving them. But he said, "I must proclaim the good news of the kingdom of God to the other towns also, because that is why I was sent." And he kept on preaching in the synagogues of Judea.

Luke 4:42–44

TODAY'S THOUGHT:

In the 21st century, a perception has been created by society for the need to do more, see more, be more. You are asked to help coach the little league team, help out with an additional project at work, volunteer with another organization, the list goes on and on. There is almost a pressure, so you aren't viewed as lazy, to fill up your calendar completely and then squeeze in an additional commitment.

In this process, you may have abandoned one of the most useful words for keeping your sanity...the word "*no.*" The word "*yes*" has become the default answer, when it should only be reserved for certain times. If we break it down and examine it, there are a lot of reasons why we find ourselves saying "*yes,*" even when it's not best. We feel the pressure to try to please everyone. We want to make our friends happy. We want to fit in. We want to impress our boss or co-workers. We want to grow in the company and get promoted. We want to be noticed as a top student. We want our life to appear as one that has it all together. So, we end up increasing the pace of our life by saying "*yes*" too often.

The reality is when you say YES to something, you are saying NO to something else.[18] Many times, you end up saying "*no*" to your mental health and that's a dangerous path to go down. Scripture makes it crystal clear that Jesus said "*no*" often. Even 2,000 years ago, Jesus knew when he said YES to something, he would be saying NO to something else. As George Niederauer said, "*Jesus said 'no' when a 'yes' did not fit in with His 'yes' to the Father.*"[19] There is tremendous power in learning to say "*no.*" In each situation, you may have to ask yourself, "If I do this, what will I not be able to do as result or what will I be sacrificing?" And then ask, "What is more important?" Just like Jesus did, you may have to say "*no*" to something good, so you can say "*yes*" to something of greater value. Make your "*yes*" the exception, not the rule.

QUESTIONS TO CONSIDER:

- Is your default answer usually "*yes?*" Why do you think you have trouble saying "*no?*"

- What kind of requests, activities, events, do you need to start saying "*no*" to?

TAKEAWAY:

Identify what you have the bandwidth for and then rank the most valuable components of your life. Any other invitation or request beyond that can only be responded to with a "*yes*" if you are able to fit it in or replace it with something else.

---

[18] https://www.brainyquote.com/quotes/sean_covey_657207
[19] Donald J. Hying, "Questions to Ponder as We Enter into the Forty Days of Lent," *NWI Catholic,* accessed October 15, 2020,
https://www.nwicatholic.com/index.php/2011-10-28-15-52-16/bishop-hying-col umn/3408-questions-to-ponder-as-we-enter-into-the-forty-days-of-lent.

DAY 39: JOY, JOY, JOY

GOD'S WORD:

Finally, brothers and sisters, whatever is true, whatever is noble, whatever is right, whatever is pure, whatever is lovely, whatever is admirable—if anything is excellent or praiseworthy—think about such things.

Philippians 4:8

TODAY'S THOUGHT:

I drive a 2004 Jeep, so I don't have any of the fancy features that my wife has in the vehicle she drives. Many of these features are safety features, designed to help protect the driver and the car. The one that comes to mind is the tiny camera, near the bumper, that allows the driver to see what is directly behind the car when reversing. Also, the car will make a beeping noise when it gets a certain distance from another object, warning the driver to stop. I could say that my old Jeep makes a noise as well, but sadly, the sound would be from crashing into another object. The camera and the beeping noise are signs of potential danger. The driver then has the choice to either listen to the beeping and believe what the camera is displaying, or to ignore it and face the consequences.

Every day, you have a similar situation that takes place in your life. A war is raging in the battlefield of your mind. Your thoughts hold tremendous potential to either improve or destroy your life. They have the power to help lift you up or drag you down. What you allow to come into your mind, and, more importantly, stay in your mind, dictates the quality of your life. Satan will do everything in his power to have you focus on negativity. He knows if you focus on negativity long enough, it will rob you of your joy. You cannot always dictate what enters your mind, but you do have control over what stays.

Luckily, believers have the best warning system...the Holy Spirit. In the same way that a vehicle's safety features warn of danger, as wrong thoughts start to enter your mind, the Holy Spirit prompts and convicts you. The beeping is loud and evident. But God gives you free will. You make the choice to listen to the warnings or to ignore them. As you choose to listen to the warning signs, you are able to spot lies from Satan and identify the thoughts that are not of God. Then, instead of allowing those lies to occupy your mind, you *reject* them and *replace* them. You replace them with truths of God that lead to joy. Satan is no match for the Word of God. *Pick up your sword and head into the battlefield for your mind!*

QUESTIONS TO CONSIDER:

- Are there people, shows, music, activities that feed your mind with wrong thoughts? Mentally list them. (The larger the quantity of wrong or evil thoughts that enter your mind, the harder it is to clean it out, which leads to less space for right thinking.)

- If the answer is yes, will you decide to limit or distance yourself completely from it?

TAKEAWAY:

Say this prayer: Lord, I want to focus on right thinking that leads to joy. Help me identify thoughts that are not from You and replace them with thoughts that are. Amen.

DAY 40: TAKING REFUGE

GOD'S WORD:

*Have mercy on me, my God, have mercy on me, for in you I take refuge. I
will take refuge in the shadow of your wings until the disaster has passed.*

Psalms 57:1

TODAY'S THOUGHT:

David wrote Psalm 57 while he was in a cave, playing the deadliest
game of hide and seek. David was doing the hiding and Saul, who
wanted to take David's life, was doing the seeking. David was in the
cave scared, confused, uncertain if he would survive to see another
day. It was in those moments of fear that he realized his need to run
to the shadow of God's wings, because there he would find refuge.
Re-read Psalm 57:1 with that context in mind. Pretty powerful, right?

When my daughter, Juliette, was a toddler, there was a severe
storm with loud thunder and bright lightning. The storm startled
Juliette so much that she jumped up from the toys she was playing
with and ran in my direction. As she sprinted towards me, she said,
"I want to take refuge in your arms until the thunder stops." I guess
it wasn't quite in those words; she was just a toddler. It was closer
to, *"Daddy, help me!"* Juliette understood the storm was happening
all around her and it left her scared. But as soon as she ran into her
daddy's arms, she felt comforted. She felt safe. The storm was still
going on, but she trusted that I would take care of her until it stopped.

Through the storm of mental illness or a dangerous game of hide
and seek, you can take refuge in the arms of God. You can run to God
to find the peace and comfort that you so desperately desire. Fear,
confusion, uncertainty will try to call the shots, but they do not have

to loom over your life. You can make the choice to override those emotions and look to God. Refuge can be found in Him, whether the storm lasts a season or for the rest of your life.

QUESTIONS TO CONSIDER:

- What is it, in or around your life, that leads you to the cave, scared and confused? Why is that?
- Should it have crippling power over you?
- Will you decide to run to the arms of God for refuge instead?

TAKEAWAY:

Say this prayer: God, I do not understand what is going on in my life. I am scared. I worry I will not be able to make it, but I know it is not dependent on my power or strength. I will run to Your arms to find refuge until the storm has passed. Thank You for providing shelter for me. Amen.

DAY 41: PEACE OF GOD

GOD'S WORD:

Peace I leave with you; my peace I give you. I do not give to you as the world gives. Do not let your hearts be troubled and do not be afraid.

John 14:27

TODAY'S THOUGHT:

When battling mental illness, all you want is a little peace, and if you are honest, some days it's nowhere to be found. No matter what you do or say; no matter where you are, peace appears to be non-existent. Today's verse shows that peace is always available, because it has been promised by God. It is available in the high and low moments of life. True peace is provided by God, but you play a role in the receiving of peace. It takes you being intentional, seeking Christ, and not hindering the peace of God to fill your life.

That sounds good, but what does that actually mean? Let's break it down. Your thoughts dictate the quality of your life. What often happens is that we give our attention to our emotions instead, living life and making decisions based off of feelings. If there is anything I know about emotions and feelings, it is that they constantly change. Feelings, with no support system, are one of the most inconsistent things in life. You can't rely on something inconsistent to be the basis for decision-making. Your feelings should never dictate your thinking.

Here's why that is so important to realize: whatever you focus on, you tend to walk towards and begin to follow. Since your mind can only focus on one thing at a time, if you focus on a lie, chances are that you will buy into the lie, and walk in the way of that lie. Wrong thinking always leads to wrong feeling and to bad decision-making. RIGHT thinking should dictate your feelings. You are to think on, take hold of, focus on the things of Christ, until your mind is renewed. When you are focused on the things of God, when your mind is renewed, then you will feel the peace of God covering you.

QUESTIONS TO CONSIDER:

- Are there things in your life (people, shows, music, activities) that feed your mind with wrong thoughts? We can't block all of it necessarily, but we usually can filter out quite a bit.

- Which of these things do you need to step away from to some degree?

- What can you do to fill your mind with the things of Christ?

TAKEAWAY:

Say this prayer: God, I need Your peace in my life. I know I can't achieve peace alone. But I also know that I play a role in choosing what enters my mind. I choose to focus on You today. Amen.

DAY 42: I WORRY THAT I WORRY TOO MUCH

GOD'S WORD:

Do not be anxious about anything, but in every situation, by prayer and petition, with thanksgiving, present your requests to God. And the peace of God, which transcends all understanding, will guard your hearts and your minds in Christ Jesus.

Philippians 4:6–7

TODAY'S THOUGHT:

When my daughter, Juliette, was a toddler, she would always want to hand her trash to me, and she would keep her eyes on me until it was thrown away. Even at that age, she was extremely observant and could spot trash anywhere, at any time. Once she saw the trash, she could not rest or enjoy what we were doing, until she knew that it had been properly disposed of. After repeatedly seeing me take the trash from her and put it in the trashcan, she began to trust that, as long as she got the trash to Daddy, it would be thrown away. From then on, I always found it fascinating; the moment I would stick out my hand and take the trash from her, I could sense the stress and worry leave her body and mind. I hadn't thrown the trash away yet, but she knew that she did not have to worry about it anymore; Daddy would take care of it.

Every day in your life, there will be opportunities to worry about finances, relationships, work, school, health, uncertainty with the future, and so on. As a result, worry can become a regular aspect of your life. The Greek word of *"worry"* is translated *"to be pulled in different directions.*" That is what worry feels like. I am sure you know how that feels. It's not healthy, and it most definitely takes a toll on your mental health.

Paul shares in today's verses that God desires to take your anxiety and worry and replace them with peace. Instead of putting all of the pressure on yourself to think through every possible scenario or fix the issue, God wants you to approach Him in prayer and ask Him to help you figure it out. God wants to move you from *worry* to *peace*. Engaging with God in prayer does not mean that the scenario in front of you will be resolved like magic, but it does allow you to have peace in the midst of the scenario. Just like when Juliette handed me trash; even though the trash had not been thrown away yet, she didn't have to worry anymore. Daddy would take care of it.

Hand the worry to God, keep working hard with what is in front of you, but leave the results in God's hands. Follow what Martin Luther said, *"Pray, and let God worry."*[20]

Questions To Consider:

- Do you tend to try and fix everything yourself? Do you struggle with letting go? If so, why do you think that is your tendency?

- Just imagine if you were to truly trust God with the results; what kind of peace would that bring to your life?

Takeaway:

Say this prayer: God, I have been worrying myself sick, thinking everything is on my shoulders. I want to hand that worry to You. Your Word says that You will hand peace back in exchange. I need that in my life right now. Amen.

---

[20] "Martin Luther Quotes," *Brainy Quotes*, Accessed September 25, 2020, https://www.brainyquote.com/quotes/martin_luther_151431.

DAY 43: IS PAIN A WASTE?

GOD'S WORD:

When the foundations are being destroyed, what can the righteous do? The Lord is in his holy temple; the Lord is on his heavenly throne.

Psalms 11:3–4

TODAY'S THOUGHT:

Your mind can convince you that your suffering has no purpose and your pain is a complete waste. It's rather easy to get sucked into that train of thought. Over the next few days, I want you to focus on the truth that your pain is not a waste; but rather, it is something useful.

Jesus knows what it's like to suffer, just like you and me. He endured pain in a way that we can't even come close to comprehending. Looking at the life, death, and resurrection of Jesus, because He is the example we strive to follow, it's evident that Jesus' pain was definitely not a waste. God took the worst Friday in history, when Jesus died on the cross for our sins, and turned it into the most victorious Sunday, when Jesus rose from the dead and defeated sin and death. The greatest purpose came out of Jesus' worst pain.

King David explained in Psalms 11:3–4 that when chaos and pain surround you, this is what you can do...know and believe that God is still good, and that God is still on His throne. You can't dictate what pain you will experience, but you determine your perspective and how you will respond. Following God doesn't stop life's hardships or pain from coming, but you can believe in your spirit that God can be trusted and that He is doing what is best for you. Enlarge your concept of God.

Questions To Consider:

- What kind of pain have you dealt with in your life?

- Even though you have experienced pain in the past and seen God come through, why is it so difficult to see any purpose while in the midst of new pain?

- Does it bring any comfort knowing that Jesus actually understands what it is like to suffer and feel pain? How so?

Takeaway:

Write out the verse for today, Psalms 11:3–4 and read it at least five times throughout the day.

DAY 44: CREATED FOR THE VALLEY

GOD'S WORD:

Consider it pure joy, my brothers and sisters, whenever you face trials of many kinds, because you know that the testing of your faith produces perseverance. Let perseverance finish its work so that you may be mature and complete, not lacking anything.

James 1:2–4

TODAY'S THOUGHT:

Oh, how nice it would be to always stay on the mountaintop, where there seems to be no trouble or heartaches; only beauty and a nice breeze. We don't want to go down to the valley. It's painful. It's scary. It's overwhelming. But we have no choice over the matter, and it is a good thing that we don't. Staying on the mountaintop wouldn't be best for you. You don't learn and grow on the mountaintop. You're not as teachable on the mountaintop because life is cruising. You don't really see the need to examine your life or slow down to ask God for guidance.

But in the valley experiences, the toughest times in your life, you have the opportunity to grow at a tremendous rate. It's in those moments when you are running low on strength, when life's circumstances are beyond your comprehension; that you are left with two options...*you panic, or you pray.* When you lean into God, your character is being built. The testing of your faith, the trial, the hardship, the pain produces perseverance. Perseverance, or another word, endurance, is a growing determination in the face of adversity, based on hope. Or a shorter definition is: *Perseverance is victory over trial.* The pain, the suffering leads to a determination to get through it; to push through the pain until victory. Through perseverance, facing adversity and getting through it, something amazing happens....it matures you in Christ. It produces godly character in you.

God uses your suffering, pain, and hardships to grow you. What you are enduring is not a waste. When you are most vulnerable, you are the most teachable. You learn more in your valley experiences than your mountaintops. If you are in the valley right now, know that God is working on you and making you more like Him!

QUESTIONS TO CONSIDER:

- Can you think of a time (maybe you are in one right now) where you got to a place of panic or pray? How did you handle the situation? What did you choose?

- What character traits in your life have you already seen grow over the years? What traits need to be worked on next?

TAKEAWAY:

Say this prayer: Lord, I am going to choose to be thankful for the seasons in the valley, because I know it is growing me. Use those times to mold me into the follower of Christ You want me to be. Amen.

DAY 45: USEFULNESS THROUGH BROKENNESS

GOD'S WORD:

Praise be to the God and Father of our Lord Jesus Christ, the Father of compassion and the God of all comfort, who comforts us in all our troubles, so that we can comfort those in any trouble with the comfort we ourselves receive from God. For just as we share abundantly in the sufferings of Christ, so also our comfort abounds through Christ.

2 Corinthians 1:3–5

TODAY'S THOUGHT:

Paul, the author of Corinthians, wrote about a thorn in his side, some type of battle or struggle he was never able to get rid of. Paul wanted deliverance from this weakness; he wanted a substitution. But God's plan was not for him to have a substitution, but to have transformation instead. As Paul relied on the power of God in his weakest moments, God transformed the life of Paul and expanded the Kingdom of God through Paul in ways that Paul would have never imagined. Paul's life and teachings show you and me that there is usefulness through brokenness. There is something powerful that happens as you walk through difficulties and keep your eyes on Christ. The more broken you are, the more you are able to rely on the power and strength of God. Not only does it grow your character, but your life becomes an example of the power of God to the people around you. You have the opportunity to help people that you may not have had without the thorn or hardship.

Charles Stanley said, *"Brokenness is God's requirement for maximum usefulness."*[21] This is evident throughout the entire Bible. The most broken people make the biggest waves for the gospel. The trial, the mental illness, was allowed in your life for an eternal reason – a purpose beyond what you can see or understand at the moment. God will use it for your ultimate good (perhaps in ways you may never understand) and the good of His Kingdom, if you trust and submit it to Him.

If you can look at your pain, hardships, mental illness as an opportunity to bring out your sufficiency in Christ and showcase His divine grace, it will help sustain your soul and give you the ability to praise God, even in the deepest, darkest valleys. Instead of asking, *"How can I get out of this mess?"* Begin asking, *"How can God be glorified in this situation?"*

Questions To Consider:

- How might God want to use your pain and hardships to comfort the people He has placed in front of you?

- What can you do to make sure that you are being intentional to see the opportunities to share your faith?

Takeaway:

Say this prayer: Lord, use my brokenness for Your glory. It hurts, it's hard to understand, but I know You are working. I know You will use it for my good and for the good of Your Kingdom. Amen.

---

[21] Charles Stanley, *30 Life Principles* (Atlanta: Touch Ministries, 2008), 77.

DAY 46: THE SUN STILL SHINES

GOD'S WORD:

For it is God who works in you to will and to act
in order to fulfill his good purpose.

Philippians 2:13

TODAY'S THOUGHT:

Even when the clouds are blocking the sun, the sun still shines. It still provides energy that the plants need for photosynthesis. It still balances out the elements so that earth doesn't freeze over. It still causes skin to burn. Just because it may not be shining as bright or because you can't feel the heat as much as on a cloudless day, it does not mean the sun has stopped doing what it does.

God is working even when your life seems to have a cloud above it. Even when life is not going as planned. Even when there is uncertainty. Just because you may not see the way that God is working in the moment, does not mean that He is not. You may ask, "But what about my depression?" God is in the middle of it with you. "What about my anxiety?" God is not surprised or overwhelmed by it. "What about my Obsessive-Compulsive Disorder?" God is working. "What about my Bipolar Disorder?" God is not limited. "What about my Post-Traumatic Stress Disorder?" God is in control.

Even when you cannot feel it, God is working things out for your good and the good of His Kingdom. Life's circumstances cannot stop God from doing what He does. Lean into that truth today and be confident that God is not only big enough to be working, but that He also cares about you enough to provide everything you need.

Questions To Consider:

- Are you at a place in your life where it feels like God is not working in, around, or through you? If so, what is the main cause of that?

- What can you do this week to remind yourself that God is indeed working and will continue to work in your life?

Takeaway:

Listen to the song "Way Maker"[22] by Leeland at some point today. Let the bridge of the song, written out below, be the cry of your heart.

Even when I don't see it, You're working.
Even when I don't feel it, You're working.
You never stop, You never stop working.
You never stop, You never stop working.

---

[22] Leeland Mooring, "Way Maker," *Better Word*, Integrity Music, 2019. *Youtube,* youtube.com/watch?v=iJCV_2H9xD0.

DAY 47: FIGHT OR FLIGHT

GOD'S WORD:

I have told you these things, so that in me you may have peace. In this world you will have trouble. But take heart! I have overcome the world.

John 16:33

TODAY'S THOUGHT:

Imagine you are in the aquarium tank at Sea World and you realize there is a Great White Shark swimming underneath you. What happens when you realize the shark is in the tank with you? You wouldn't start texting some friends back or eating candy! Your mind would immediately concentrate on one thing and one thing only...is this going to be fight or flight? You know you need to either stay in the tank and fight, or you need get out of the tank before the shark attacks.

Kendra Cherry, author and educator, explained it as, *"The fight-or-flight response (also known as the acute stress response), refers to a physiological reaction that occurs when we are in the presence of something that is mentally or physically terrifying."*[23]

For you, you have a fight or flight mode based off of certain circumstances. When it gets to that place, there is a pausing point, where you decide which option you are going with. During that period, there can be an increase in blood pressure, heart rate, and your breathing rate. Fight or flight response can be triggered by

---

[23]Kendra Cherry, "How the Fight-or-Flight Response Works," *Very Well Mind.* Updated August 18, 2019,
https://www.verywellmind.com/what-is-the-fight-or-flight-response-2795194.

something that is a real threat or even one that is imaginary. The key aspect is that your mind believes it is real.

It is crucially important that you do everything you can to pre-plan and post-observe for better understanding. When you find yourself getting to a place of fight or flight, try to identify what exactly it is that is causing you to become tense. For someone that is extremely anxious about flying in an airplane, for example, the foundational reason for the anxiety can be a number of things: a need for control, claustrophobia, fear of flights.

You have to examine, perhaps talk with someone else, and do some research to figure out what exactly is causing you to panic and run away out of fear. Once you can identify that, it's much easier to learn ways to calm down your mind and body when you do get worked up. Identify a scripture passage that specifically addresses that fear and quote it in the moment. The Word of God has the ability to transform and renew our minds.

Let's limit the amount of unnecessary fight or flight moments you have and then determine how you will fight against it when it does come. You can rest assured that God will give you the strength that you need because He already overcame the world.

QUESTIONS TO CONSIDER:

- What is your flight cue? What is it you are running from exactly? What is the core reason?

- How can you put yourself in a position to allow God to give you the strength that you need in those moments?

TAKEAWAY:

Take at least 10 minutes to think and write down your answers for these questions. As you answer this, be aware that there may be additional layers. If your answer is a need for control, you can peel it back and see more detail of why you feel that need and what is causing it.

DAY 48: NEVER-ENDING SUPPLY

GOD'S WORD:

Yet this I call to mind and therefore I have hope: Because of the LORD's great love we are not consumed, for his compassions never fail. They are new every morning; great is your faithfulness.

Lamentations 3:21–23

TODAY'S THOUGHT:

I have an electric weed-eater that I use when taking care of the yard. Every time I use it, I feel as if I'm going to lose my mind. My front and backyard are both rather small, but the weed-eater only has enough battery for me to finish the front yard. I then go and plug it in to charge, hoping to use it again soon, but it requires quite some time before it has enough juice to finish the backyard. I'm getting frustrated just writing this right now! It shouldn't bother me this much, but I always wonder why it couldn't have been made in a way where the power supply didn't run out so quickly. And no, this is not my attempt of sending out an S.O.S for someone to mail me a new weed-eater.

I write this because you and I experience this feeling in life with way more than just weed-eaters. You might run out of energy multiple times daily, or experience highs and lows within a couple of days, or you fall short and wonder if you have messed up one too many times. And you question if your power supply is able to make it to the "backyard" of the day or of your life.

Every single person, especially those with mental illness, need the confidence of a never-ending supply. The confidence of knowing you will have what you need, when you need it, however you need it. That is something we cannot supply or promise ourselves in our power. It requires the presence of God. Luckily for us, because of God's character, He is unable to be unfaithful. Being faithful is a part of who God is. The verse for today shares that the river of His mercy never runs dry. Every morning, God gives a fresh supply of compassion and love to us. Nothing or no one else has the capability to come through for you all of the time. Your job can't. Any earthly relationship can't. Success can't. In a world that constantly changes and lets you down, only God is fully faithful. The thought of this limitless supply that God will offer every single day should overwhelm us, leaving our response as, *"Great is Your faithfulness!"*

QUESTIONS TO CONSIDER:

- God has new mercies for you every single day. What if you actually, fully believed that?

- How would that change your perspective?

- Will you choose to believe that today?

TAKEAWAY:

Write down, on a piece of paper or index card, a handful of words of something that stood out to you from the reading: something God highlighted for you. Place it somewhere you will see it throughout the next few days. For example, you can write something like:

- Lamentations 3:22–23 – God's compassions never fail

- New mercy

- Great is Your faithfulness.

- Get Jared a new weed-eater. (Totally kidding!)

DAY 49: FIRM FOUNDATION

GOD'S WORD:

Therefore everyone who hears these words of mine and puts them into practice is like a wise man who built his house on the rock. The rain came down, the streams rose, and the winds blew and beat against that house; yet it did not fall, because it had its foundation on the rock. But everyone who hears these words of mine and does not put them into practice is like a foolish man who built his house on sand. The rain came down, the streams rose, and the winds blew and beat against that house, and it fell with a great crash.

Matthew 7:24–27

TODAY'S THOUGHT:

Recently, we have dealt with foundation issues; the dreaded nightmare of being a homeowner. If you have ever dealt with your house's foundation, I connect with you on a deep level and feel your pain. At first, we only noticed a small crack here and there. But slowly those cracks grew and then one day; BAM...a large crack surfaced from one end of the house to the other. We knew we were in trouble. For months, I was on the phone with the insurance company and foundation repair and plumbing companies. If we did not take the necessary steps to fix and secure our house, it would continue to face the consequences. The foundation affects everything about the house.

Jesus talks about building your house, your life, on a firm foundation. In the verses before today's passage, Jesus had just finished giving the Sermon on the Mount, which was a message about doing, not just thinking or believing. He explained that it is one thing to hear something and another to apply it to your life. Adding onto that message, Jesus showed that the house stood firm because those living in the house knew what to do and actually did it; they built upon a rock. Your life's foundation becomes stronger and more secure as your faith grows. Your faith grows from learning about God and applying what you learn to your life. There are two sides to this, though. Simply hearing or knowing, but not doing and putting into practice, is foolishness. That is like a house that, when the storms come, when hardships surround you, when life continues to take a toll on your mental health, when you face financial obstacles, when your faith is tested, when you feel rejected or wronged, the house can only withstand the storm to a certain extent before it comes crashing down. Then you are left feeling hopeless, uncertain if you can continue on, unsure if God really cares.[24]

I do not want that for your life. You need a firm foundation. Your mental health needs it. Your relationships need it. Your sense of security and purpose needs it. Everything about your life desperately needs it. Take what you read in the Bible and apply it your life. Allow your foundation to grow stronger. Then you will have confidence that your house can withstand the storms of life.

QUESTIONS TO CONSIDER:

- Examine your life: how much of your foundation is grounded in you and how much in God?

- What is one thing you have learned about God recently that you can apply to your life?

TAKEAWAY:

This may sound elementary but give it a try. Take a piece of paper and draw a simple house. Underneath the house, draw a large rectangle, which will signify the foundation. Inside the foundation, write out some of the things you have learned from God's Word. That could include His attributes (love, wisdom, faithfulness, etc.), the teachings

---

[24] Andy Stanley, "Big Life," Grow Up Series. Orange Curriculum: The reThink Group, 2010.

of Jesus, truths about who you are and how you are to live. After you finish that, write inside of the house, "My house is built on the solid foundation of God."

Your life's foundation becomes stronger
and more secure as your faith grows.

DAY 50: CUT YOURSELF SOME SLACK

GOD'S WORD:

*I lift up my eyes to the mountains— where does my help come from? My
help comes from the LORD, the Maker of heaven and earth.*

Psalms 121:1–2

TODAY'S THOUGHT:

There are some nights that my wife and I finally get the girls to bed
(we had no idea bedtime would be so exhausting and drawn out) and
I sit down on the couch and think, *"I am not cut out for this. I can't
do this whole parenting thing."* I want to always show consistency,
display love and grace, handle situations and shortcomings as teaching opportunities, but there are a lot of days that I feel I fall short
from completing every single one of those. My wife has to remind
me regularly that I am a good father and give the girls more than
they could ask for. I think the struggle for me is the expectations I
set for myself, because at times, the level I expect is perfection.

If you are anything like me, you overthink way too much...at
home, work, school, writing emails, sending texts, when you're with
friends or family. It can raise your anxiety, stress you out, leave you
feeling defeated, because no one has the capability to be perfect. God
doesn't even want your aim to be perfection. He simply asks you
to work hard with what He has given you and to love Him and love
others.

So, remind yourself as often as you need that you aren't called to
be a perfect parent, student, employee, boss, spouse, friend. You are
called to look to the perfect God and keep your eyes on Him. When
you do fall short, you get back up and give it another try. When you

aren't sure if you did enough or if you are enough, know that God doesn't see you in that way. When He looks at you, He sees His child. You are enough because you are His.

QUESTIONS TO CONSIDER:

- Do you aim for perfection too often? In what way?

- In what area do you need to cut yourself some slack?

TAKEAWAY:

Say this prayer: Lord, I will keep my eyes on You and be faithful to love and care for the people You have placed in my life. I will leave my approval in Your hands. Amen.

DAY 51: COMPARISON TRAP

GOD'S WORD:

And I saw that all toil and all achievement spring from one person's envy of another. This too is meaningless, a chasing after the wind.

Ecclesiastes 4:4

TODAY'S THOUGHT:

There are tons of traps out in the world. One of the worst traps people can get caught in is the trap of comparison. Looking at your life, you may say that you've had seasons or instances where you could not stop from comparing yourself to others and what they were doing and achieving. Social media has tremendously multiplied this happening. Now, more people's lives are put in front of you and you are being fed their highlight reel. It is similar to the top ten plays on sport channels. They post their best moments, with their best stuff, when they look their best. Who wants to post a bad angle of them eating Cheetos?

King Solomon addressed the tendency to compare yourself to other people. He said it is like someone running around trying to catch the wind, which could never happen. That is how comparison is. There is never a sense of satisfaction. The deeper you fall into this trap, the steeper the uphill battle becomes with your mental illness. You either place unnecessary pressure on yourself in an effort to "catch" someone else, or you think less of yourself. Neither is the right option. There is absolutely NO win in comparison.

Instead of focusing on what others have that you don't, ask God to help you see and enjoy what He has blessed YOU with. If you continue to focus on this, God will begin to change your perspective.

Questions To Consider:

- When do you find yourself most tempted to compare? On social media? With certain people? In certain places?

- What would happen if you began to let go of comparisons? What might be the result?

Takeaway:

Say this prayer: God, I want to focus on what You have given me. Thank You for my talents, passions, gifts, and the people You have placed around me. Most importantly, thank You for loving me. Amen.

DAY 52: THE MEASURING STICK

GOD'S WORD:

Yet to all who did receive him, to those who believed in his name, he gave the right to become children of God
John 1:12

TODAY'S THOUGHT:

A yardstick is a stick that is one yard (crazy how I figured that one out), which is 3 feet. The yardstick is one of the tools used to measure. Even in elementary school, kids start using rulers and learning how inches and centimeters work. After you use a ruler, a yardstick, a tape measure, you can be confident that what you just measured is correct. Whether you are measuring wood, seeing how much your toddler has grown, or seeing how far you can spit, you can feel secure. When it comes to your life and wanting to know if you are doing okay, what are you using as your measuring stick? What are you using to see your worth? You will look somewhere to determine if you are a good enough spouse, child, parent, worker, student, athlete, human being.

When my depression and anxiety worsen, I tend to struggle with my identity and if I am enough. As we saw yesterday, if we're not careful, we can look to people and places to see if we measure up, and every single one of them is not qualified to give us an answer. The only One powerful enough to answer that is God. When I ask if I measure up, God answers by telling me that because I accepted His free gift of salvation, I am His child. That quickly answers if I am enough. As a child of God, I have more than anything this world could offer.

When you wonder if you are enough or if you are doing okay in life, look to God and trust His answer. His answer is the only one that matters. Allow God to be your measuring stick.

Questions To Consider:

- What are you using as your measuring stick to find validation, value, and acceptance?

- Do you find yourself turning to other things around you? Job, people, achievements?

- Have you accepted God's gift of salvation? If not, I believe it's the greatest decision you can ever make. Refer back to Day 11 where I walk through how to do this.

Takeaway:

Say this prayer: God, I do not want to fall into the trap of comparison. Please help me to not allow other people's achievements or status to be my measuring stick. I will find my worth in You. I will find my validation in You. Amen.

DAY 53: WORKMANSHIP

GOD'S WORD:

For we are God's workmanship, created in Christ Jesus to do good works,
which God prepared in advance for us to do.

Ephesians 2:10

TODAY'S THOUGHT:

There may be days where you watch a movie, see an Instagram post, or watch a music video and think about these "cool" opportunities some people have in life. *"Some people have it all and get to experience life in a way I never will"* may be your thought. It appears they have it all and don't have to suffer in the way you know you do. You may feel limited because of your journey with mental illness. It is easy to get caught in this mindset. What is deceiving, though, is that you and I have NO idea what other people are going through. Sometimes we don't even truly know what our friends are experiencing, so there is no way to know what a celebrity or someone we've seen from a distance is battling.

Just because they may have some bright moments in their lives, does not mean that their lives are of more value and worth than your life. They are not more special than you and I. The danger in that thought process is it's actually pointing the finger at God, claiming He messed up when He created you; that He didn't do a good enough job. Who are we to critique the Creator of the magnificent universe we see around us?

Ephesians 2:10 explains how valuable you are. The Greek word translated *"workmanship"* is the word *"poema,"* which is where we

117

get our word for poetry. You have value, not because you worked for that, but because God pieced you together. You are God's poetry. His workmanship. His poem. Because you are the artwork of God, you have extreme value. God makes no mistakes. He intentionally distributed to each person certain gifts, talents, and opportunities. While you may be limited in one aspect with mental illness, God wired you with a specific skill set or opportunity that others don't have. Without you using those, the world would miss out. Celebrate the gifts God gave you. Focus on being who God created you to be, work hard with the opportunities He places in front of you, and leave the results up to Him.

QUESTIONS TO CONSIDER:

- Do you tend to look at the life of others and compare what they appear to have to what you don't?

- If you were to focus on being who God has called you to be, how would it affect your relationships? Your job? School? Outlook on life?

TAKEAWAY:

Take time to write out specific gifts, talents, skills God gave you. (This is only for you to see, so do not worry about being humble.) After you make the list, pray to God, thanking Him for each one and then ask how He wants to use those to bring others to Him.

DAY 54: EXPAND MY HORIZON

GOD'S WORD:

Jabez cried out to the God of Israel, "Oh, that you would bless me and enlarge my territory! Let your hand be with me, and keep me from harm so that I will be free from pain." And God granted his request.

1 Chronicles 4:10

TODAY'S THOUGHT:

For the next two days, I want to focus on a famous prayer that is recorded in the Old Testament called *The Prayer of Jabez*. It is a powerful prayer with numerous nuggets of truth packed into it. My hope is that this becomes a prayer that you and I begin praying for ourselves on a regular basis. As Jabez prayed to God, the first thing he asked was that God would bless him. This can seem like a strange request, because we think of blessings as a greedy desire to receive more of what we want. In the Bible, to ask for blessings from God was to ask for God's supernatural favor. Bruce Wilkinson explains that, *"When we ask God's blessing, we're not asking for more of what we could get for ourselves. We're crying out for the wonderful, unlimited goodness that only God has the power to know about or give to us."*[25] It is a request to be equipped with what God wanted to give him. Have you ever prayed that God would give you exactly what you needed, nothing more, nothing less?

My favorite aspect of this verse is the next request. When Jabez called out to God to enlarge his territory, he did not do this out of

---

[25] Bruce Wilkinson, *Prayer of Jabez* (Sisters, Oregon: Multnomah Publishers, Inc., 2000), 23.

selfish ambition. He did not hope to be famous for popularity. His aim was not wealth or possessions. Jabez desired for God to enlarge his life and his realm of influence, so that he could bring greater glory to God. He wanted to make as big of an impact for the Kingdom of God as he could. What if you prayed that for your life? What if you desired for God to expand your horizon, influence, opportunity; not out of selfish desire, but so that you could further the gospel? My prayer in recent months has been for God to enlarge my territory for mental health awareness. I see a need for people to find Jesus in the middle of mental illness, so my desire is for God to use me in as big of a scale as He wants, to impact as many people as possible.

The world around you is a mission field. People need to see Jesus in the midst of chaos, confusion, hurt, disaster, mental illness, disease, pain. The world will see that through you as God pours His favor on you and enlarges your territory.

QUESTIONS TO CONSIDER:

- Does asking God to bless you feel strange? Does it feel selfish? Is it because you might be viewing it as an earthly blessing, not a spiritual blessing?

- God wants to bless you and enlarge your territory for His glory, not yours. What safeguards or accountability can you put into place to make sure you stay focused on the kingdom of God as He expands your horizon?

TAKEAWAY:

Say this Prayer: God, I come to You humbling myself. I ask for You to bless me, by providing Your supernatural favor. I want more of Your goodness in my life. Enlarge my territory. I want to make Your name famous. I want to make an impact for Your Kingdom. Amen.

DAY 55: THE HAND OF GOD

GOD'S WORD:

Jabez cried out to the God of Israel, "Oh, that you would bless me and enlarge my territory! Let your hand be with me, and keep me from harm so that I will be free from pain." And God granted his request.

1 Chronicles 4:10

TODAY'S THOUGHT:

Yesterday, we began examining this verse. Today, we will continue with the second part of it. The third request of Jabez was for God's divine hand to be on him. God's favor was already with him, his territory was being enlarged, now Jabez wanted to surrender his talents for God to work through him in a mighty way. He wanted God's supernatural power and presence in his life. Bruce Wilkinson said, *"You could call God's hand on you 'the touch of greatness.' You do not become great; He becomes great through you."*[26]

God has given you talents and experiences that can and should be used for His glory. There are situations, struggles, pain in this world that you feel called to be a part of the solution. You can try to help in your own power, or you can ask for the hand of God on your life; for *"the touch of greatness,"* where He works through your life in a way that only He can.

Lastly, Jabez prayed that God would keep him from anything that would tempt him to fall into sin. His desire was to flee from evil as much as he possibly could. You will not be able to get away from temptation completely; you will still be tempted; but the wise

---

[26] Ibid., 4.

strategy is to stay as far away from sin as you can. The last thing you want is for God to grant your first three requests and then for you to fall deeper in sin. God wants to help you not only fight against sin, but also to avoid it. God granted the requests of Jabez and He desires to grant yours as well, as you pray these requests with sincerity.

QUESTIONS TO CONSIDER:

- How would your perspective change if you woke up each day with the assurance that God was going to move in and through you?

- Yesterday, I shared my calling to help with mental health awareness. What has God placed on your heart and in your life to help provide encouragement, healing, or truth?

- What can you do this week to help be a part of the solution? How can you make a difference in the lives of the people that God has placed on your heart?

TAKEAWAY:

Say this prayer: God, I want Your divine hand to rest on me. Please use every part of me for Your glory. I surrender my talents, gifts, passions, experiences to You. Keep me from evil. I want to stay far away from anything that would draw me away from You. Amen.

DAY 56: BE BOLD, BE ADVENTUROUS

GOD'S WORD:

Therefore, since we have such a hope, we are very bold.

2 Corinthians 3:12

TODAY'S THOUGHT:

Anthony Storr, an English psychiatrist and author, said, *"Originality implies being bold enough to go beyond accepted norms."*[27]
   I know, without a shadow of a doubt, that you have certain passions that have led to a vision in your mind. You have a business you want to start, a degree you want to complete, a song you want to compose, a book you want to write, a podcast you want to record, a non-profit ministry you want to create, a service opportunity you want to get trained in, a new device you want to invent. I know that there is something inside of you that longs to pursue those passions and visions. God created you in that way. He gave you unique passions. Yes, they may line up and be similar to other's passions, but yours are unique to you in some way because of your personality and experiences.
   What is holding you back from pursuing them? For most people, it is fear. Fear of failure, fear of the unknown, fear of collapsing under the mental illness. While there are times that it's not wise to take a huge step if experiencing a fragile state of mental health, most of the time, the fear is unhealthy and untrue. What you want to start or get

[27] "Anthony Storr Quotes," Quote Tab, Accessed October 2, 2020, https://www.quotetab.com/quote/by-anthony-storr/originality-implies-being-bold-enough-to-go-beyond-accepted-norms.

involved in needs to happen. Lives are waiting to be changed through your vision. Hope is waiting to be restored to people as they watch you live out your passions. Your life is waiting to be more fulfilled as you pursue what God has placed inside of you. Don't allow any illness of the mind to keep you from being bold and adventurous. Don't be afraid to try new things. Don't let the fear of the unknown with your mental state keep you from pursuing dreams and passions you know you need to pursue. Be bold!

QUESTIONS TO CONSIDER:

- What passions do you have?

- What vision comes as a result of those?

- What is holding you back from pursuing it?

TAKEAWAY:

Say this prayer: God, thank You for the passions You have given me and the vision You have laid on my heart. Give me boldness and courage to pursue them. I want to honor You in all that I do. Amen.

DAY 57: THE BITTERNESS BACKPACK

GOD'S WORD:

*Be kind and compassionate to one another, forgiving each other, just as in
Christ God forgave you.*

Ephesians 4:32

TODAY'S THOUGHT:

Has someone hurt you badly? Broken your trust? To make matters
worse, did they not even try to make things right? I hope I am not
getting you fired up right now! You may convince yourself that it is
their loss, that it doesn't really affect you ...but that tends to not be
the case. If you're not careful, you end up carrying a load of anger,
frustration, and bitterness with you everywhere you go. It is like
walking with an empty backpack (which even an empty backpack
gets tiring to carry around after an extended period of time) and
everyday a heavy rock is placed inside of your backpack. Day after
day, the weight gets heavier and harder to carry. Before long you are
carrying 100 pounds of rocks and your back is sore, your shoulders
are burning from the straps, and you are forced to stop. That is a
pretty accurate description of what bitterness does in our lives.

"*Unforgiveness is choosing to stay trapped in a jail cell of bitterness,
serving time for someone else's crime.*"[28]

Bitterness is a dangerous combination with mental illness, adding
unnecessary stress and worry to your mind. It makes managing your
mental health that much harder. You can't control what the other

---

[28] "Unforgiveness," *Live Life Happy.* Updated October 4 2011,
https://livelifehappy.com/life-quotes/unforgiveness/.

person does or doesn't do. If you wait until they change or do what you wish they would, you may wait the rest of your life. That's not fair to you or your mental health.

Do what is best for you. Move on. Let go of bitterness. Don't allow unforgiveness to rob you of your peace.

Questions To Consider:

- What is the rock in your backpack that keeps getting heavier? What bitterness is building under the surface?

- Is it worth carrying around any longer?

Takeaway:

Sometimes having a tangible way of discarding your bitterness helps. That could be writing what you are angry about and then throwing it in the trash, burning it, or drawing an X through it. Get creative. Do whatever is significant and helps you make the definite step to let go.

DAY 58: THE DIVING BOARD

GOD'S WORD:

Let us hold unswervingly to the hope we profess,
for he who promised is faithful.
Hebrews 10:23

TODAY'S THOUGHT:

Can you do me a favor? Imagine a pool that has a diving board. You can dictate the size and shape of the pool and the location. Now envision yourself standing on the diving board. In my vision, I'm wearing swim trunks with flames on the side. You can borrow that design, or you have the freedom to be creative. In this picture, you represent yourself. The diving board represents your convenience, comfort, selfish desires. And the pool represents a life lived fully committed to God. You still tracking along?

There is a point in every believer's life, where the choice has to be made to jump off the diving board into the pool of fully believing and trusting who God is. This struggle exists, because it is possible to receive salvation, but still hold onto things of this world and never actually dive into the pool. The easier route is to sit on the diving board and simply stick your feet in the water. When this happens, it is because you want God, but also want to cling to worldly things. Technically, you are in the water, but are not having to face your fears and jump in completely.

The truth is that until you are fully committed, you can never experience the depth of who God is. You do not have the opportunity to experience the deep joy, peace, and purpose that is offered for those swimming in the pool. I can visualize and remember the conversations I had with God, during the season of my life that I would call my diving board moment. I had spent most of my life as a believer with just my feet in the water. I was saved and serving God. At times, I would even hang off the diving board and get half of my body in, but I was still holding onto the diving board. I couldn't let go of the security and comfort I thought I needed from things in this world. I was especially fearful because of my mental health. It's terrifying to pray, *"God, do what you want with my life. I trust you. If you want to send me to another country, if you want me to live on people's couches because my money is going other places, if you want me to work this job or that job, if you want to use my suffering to further your Kingdom, let it be."* But I finally realized, I could not fully experience God and who He is, and I couldn't be used by God fully, until I jumped in.

When you trust God's faithfulness and dive into the pool, you will realize how great a purpose God has for you. You will experience a joy and peace that nothing or no one else in the world could have ever brought. You find yourself in a position to truly help other people and further the gospel. You will be able to do all of this, in the power of God, while managing your mental health. That is how God designed your relationship with Him to be. Jump off of the diving board and see what God has in store for your life!

QUESTIONS TO CONSIDER:

- Which position are you in: standing on the diving board, sitting with feet in, or fully in the pool? If it is one of the first two options, what is holding you back? What specifically are you holding onto tightly?

- What do you need in your life or need to happen to make the decision to fully dive into the pool of who God is? Will you make that decision today?

Takeaway:

Say this prayer: God, I want to experience You fully. I want a closer, more intimate relationship with You. Give me the courage to let go of the things of this world and jump off of the diving board. I want more of You starting today. Amen.

Until you are fully committed,
you can never experience the depth of who God is.

DAY 59: THE CROSSWALK

GOD'S WORD:

*For the Spirit God gave us does not make us timid, but gives us power, love
and self-discipline. So, do not be ashamed of the testimony about our Lord
or of me his prisoner. Rather, join with me in suffering for the gospel, by
the power of God.*

2 Timothy 1:7–8

TODAY'S THOUGHT:

Picture standing at a crosswalk with a group of people, waiting for
the light to indicate you can cross. I'm going to take a shot in the
dark here and explain what takes place. I assume it is easy to follow
the instructions of *"Do not cross"* when there are cars flying by in
front of you. But the moment that there aren't cars coming and the
road is wide open for a mile, everyone starts getting antsy. People
start looking both ways and you know they are thinking, *"I could
easily make it before any cars come."* But even though ready, everyone
is waiting, because the light *does* indicate to wait and no one else
is going. No one wants to be the first one. If one person decides to
charge out, everyone's eyes get big and they take a step forward, but
usually don't commit just yet. But as soon as the second and third
person go, it's like opening the doors for the mad rush of Black Friday
shopping. At that point, everyone begins to cross.

    This is very similar to the conversation about mental illness. For
the longest time, everyone with mental illness was waiting at the
crosswalk because there was a light indicating to keep it to yourself
and not seek any help. There was a strong taboo, a nasty stigma.
Those waiting at the crosswalk knew that something wasn't right

and reaching out for help would be good, but no one wanted to be the only one to cross the crosswalk. What if I appear weak? What if people classify me as crazy? So, everyone looked around and waited and waited. But praise God, in recent years, people have had the courage to walk across the crosswalk by sharing their struggles and seeking help. Then another person crossed, and another, then a spark was lit. It is becoming a little easier to cross the crosswalk. But mental illness awareness still has a LONG way to go.

We need to go over the crosswalk together. It will take each of us doing our part. You can do this by:

1. Accepting that mental illness does not make you weak or different.

2. Talking about it with loved ones.

3. Seeking as much help from people and resources as you can.

4. Sharing your story so others do not feel alone.

I can't wait until we are able to look back and see all of the progress that was made to lose the taboo on mental health, because we all did our part to walk across the crosswalk together. Remember, God gave you a spirit of power, love, and self-discipline. That means you can join the cause with boldness.

Questions To Consider:

- Which step are you on right now? Are you ready to take the next step?

- Be creative: What avenues can you use to share your story of mental illness to reach more people?

Takeaway:

Make the commitment to take the next step on the list this week!

DAY 60: ENJOY THE JOURNEY

GOD'S WORD:

His divine power has given us everything we need for a godly life through our knowledge of him who called us by his own glory and goodness.

2 Peter 1:3

TODAY'S THOUGHT:

Although you have come to the end of this devotional book, your journey to live fully and love freely with mental illness is just beginning. The car is packed. You've gathered necessities: water, food, gas, directions, a first aid kit. You are now set for life's road trip. That doesn't mean there won't be speedbumps on the road ahead. There will be bad weather. You will have to pull over to rest and fill up your gas tank. You may get a flat tire. But you have ALL of the resources you need in Christ. If you decide every morning, to get up and align yourself with Christ, leaning into Him for the day, you will never have a shortage of strength, guidance, peace, or love.

God made life to be enjoyed, so have fun along the journey with mental illness. As my dad always told my brother and me, *"Enjoy the journey."* He meant not to wait to have fun until we reach our destination. But enjoy each step of the way. Find joy in the little, simple things of life. That is my encouragement to you. Enjoy the journey. Even if you are in the lowest of lows, in a state of extreme anxiety, in the most uncertain and confusing time of your life, the goal can still be to enjoy where you are. Having joy right now might sound impossible, but God promises to supply joy when you are on top of the mountain and when you are down in the valley.

Keep this book available, so you can go back and be reminded of the truths of God in any circumstance you may face. I have confidence that your best days are ahead of you. Thank you for going on this journey with me. We are in this together!

Questions To Consider:

- Do you find it difficult to enjoy the time you are in right now? If your perspective was tweaked or changed, do you think it would make a difference? How so?

- Who can you reach out to and tell a couple of truths God revealed to you during these past 60 days?

Takeaway:

Say this prayer: Lord, I want to live my life full of Your love. I will use the truths and Scripture from these past 60 days to keep my confidence in You. I love You. Amen.

Works Cited

"Anthony Storr Quotes." Quote Tab. Accessed October 2, 2020.
https://www.quotetab.com/quote/by-anthony-storr/originality-im
plies-being-bold-enough-to-go-beyond-accepted-norms.

"A.W. Tozer Quotes." Good Reads. Accessed November 1, 2020.
https://www.goodreads.com/author/quotes/1082290.A_W_Tozer.

"Charles Spurgeon Quotes about Purpose." AZ Quotes. Accessed
November 1, 2020.
https://www.azquotes.com/author/13978-CharlesSpurgeon/tag/pu
rpose.

Cherry, Kendra. "How the Fight-or-Flight Response Works." *Very
Well Mind.* Updated August 18, 2019.
https://www.verywellmind.com/what-is-the-fight-or-flight-respo
nse-2795194.

Clements, Ron, John Musker, Chris Williams, and Don Hall. 2016.
Moana. United States: Walt Disney Studios Motion Pictures.

Hying, Donald J. "Questions to Ponder as We Enter into the Forty
Days of Lent." *NWI Catholic.* Accessed October 15, 2020.
https://www.nwicatholic.com/index.php/2011-10-28-15-52-16/bish
op-hying-column/3408-questions-to-ponder-as-we-enter-into-the-
forty-days-of-lent.

Ingram, Chip. "What's Your First Domino?" *Rightnow Conference.*
Orlando, Florida, 2018. https://www.rightnowmedia.org/Content/
Series/294128?episode=6.

Loritts, Crawford. "The Call to Courage." Accessed October 10, 2020.
https://preachingchristos.wordpress.com/2017/03/10/the-call-to-c
ourage-by-crawford-loritts-joshua-11-9/.

"Martin Luther Quotes." *Brainy Quotes.* Accessed September 25, 2020.
https://www.brainyquote.com/quotes/martin_luther_151431.

Mooring, Leeland. "Way Maker." *Better Word.* Integrity Music, 2019. Youtube. youtube.com/watch?v =iJCV2H9xD0.

The reThink Group, Inc. "The Word of God is a Light that Directs Our Path." *XP3 On the Lot (1) Lights!* January 2008. www.xp3students.org.

"Right Answer Quotes." AZ Quotes. Accessed October 3, 2021. https://www.azquotes.com/quotes/topics/right-answers.html.

Rogers, John, Roberto Orci and Alex Kurtzman. 2007. *Transformers.* North America: DreamWorks Pictures.

Selhub, Eva MD. "Nutritional Psychiatry: Your brain on food." *Harvard Health Publishing.* last modified March 26, 2020. https://www.health.harvard.edu/blog/nutritional-psychiatry-your-brain-on-food-201511168626.

Smith, Melinda, M.A., Lawrence Robinson, and Robert Segal, M.A.. "Sleep Needs." *Help Guide.* last modified October 2020. https://www.helpguide.org/articles/sleep/sleep-needs-get-the-sle ep-you-need.htm.

Stanley, Charles. *30 Life Principles.* Atlanta: Touch Ministries, 2008.

The Office. Deedle-Dee Productions and Reveille Productions. 2005-2013.

Tomlin, Chris. "Our God." *And If Our God is For Us.* Sparrow Records, 2010. *Youtube,* youtu.be/NJpt1hSYf2o.

"Unforgiveness." *Live Life Happy.* Updated October 4 2011. https://livelifehappy.com/life-quotes/unforgiveness/.

Wiersbe, Warren. *The Wiersbe Bible Commentary,* NT. Colorado Springs: David C. Cook, 2007.

Wiersbe, Warren. *The Wiersbe Bible Commentary,* OT. Colorado Springs: David C. Cook, 2007.

Wilkinson, Bruce. *The Prayer of Jabez.* Sisters, Oregon: Multnomah Publishers, Inc., 2000.

Index

Acts
    21:11–13, 59
Agabus, 59
anxiety, 17, 18, 29, 35, 37, 49,
    57, 93, 94, 111, 115, 133
    and prayer, 38
    and thankfulness, 71
    causes, 104

Bible, 54
bitterness, 126

Cherry, Kendra, 103
1 Chronicles
    4:10, 119, 121
Colossians
    3:15, 71
1 Corinthians
    6:19, 20
    10:31, 21
    13:4–8, 41
2 Corinthians
    1:3–5, 99
    3:12, 123
    4:7–12, 9
counseling, 31, 78

depression, 14, 22, 29, 115

diet, 21, 22
    and depression, 22

Ecclesiastes
    3:4, 48
    4:4, 113
    4:9–10, 79
embarrassment, 11, 12
    dealing with, 12
endorphins, 19
entitlement, 71
Ephesians
    2:10, 117
    2:19–22, 73
    4:32, 125
exercise, 17, 19

failure, 7
fatigue, 14
    decision, 43
fear, 65
freight train mornings, 5

happiness, 25
healing, 10
Hebrews
    4:12, 53
    10:23, 127

13:5, 3, 4
hope, 36
hopelessness, 35, 78

Ingram, Chip, 51
Isaiah
    40:31, 35
    41:1, 65
isolation, 3, 11, 73
    comfort during, 4

Jabez, 119, 121
James
    1:2-4, 97
    1:5, 43
1 John
    1:9, 45
    3:1, 7
3 John
    1:2, 19
John
    1:12, 115
    9:1-3, 69
    10:10, 63
    14:27, 91
    16:33, 103

Lamentations
    3:21-23, 105
    3:22-23, 106
life's purpose, 25
love, 8, 41
Luke
    4:42-44, 85
    5:18-25, 83

Mark
    1:35, 17

6:30-31, 23
Matthew
    7:7-8, 51
    7:24-27, 107
    11:28-30, 27
Mayo Clinic, 19
moodiness, 14
morning routine, 17
motivation
    lack of, 14

Paul, 59
perseverance, 97
1 Peter
    5:7, 37
2 Peter
    1:3, 133
Philippians
    1:12-14, 29
    2:13, 101
    3:12, 11
    4:6-7, 93
    4:8, 87
Proverbs
    11:14, 31
Psalms
    4:8, 13
    11:3-4, 95, 96
    29:11, 49
    46:10, 39
    56:8, 47
    57:1, 89
    63:3-8, 33
    100:1-5, 72
    103:12, 46
    113:1-3, 81
    119:11, 57

119:105, 55
121:1–2, 111
139:13–14, 77
145:18, 5

rest, 13, 14
rhythms, 14, 17
Romans
    5:8, 26
    6:23, 25
    10:9–10, 25
    15:13, 58

salvation, 26, 45
Scripture
    memorizing, 57
serotonin, 19
sleep, 14, 17, 19
social media, 7, 23, 113, 114
society's standards, 7, 85
strength, 5
stress, 14, 17, 21

2 Timothy
    1:7–8, 131
Tozer, A.W., 51

Wiersbe, Warren, 10, 81
worship, 33, 82
    music, 84

Made in the USA
Coppell, TX
22 August 2021